PSYCHOLOGY LIBRARY EDITIONS:
PSYCHOLINGUISTICS

Volume 5

AF705252

BILINGUALISM AND LANGUAGE DISABILITY

BILINGUALISM AND LANGUAGE DISABILITY

Assessment & Remediation

Edited by
NICK MILLER

Routledge
Taylor & Francis Group
LONDON AND NEW YORK

First published in 1984

Published 2014 by Psychology Press

Published 2016 by Routledge
2 Park Square, Milton Park, Abingdon, Oxfordshire OX14 4RN
711 Third Avenue, New York, NY 10017, USA

First issued in paperback 2015

Routledge is an imprint of the Taylor and Francis Group, an informa business

© 1984 Niklas Miller

All rights reserved. No part of this book may be reprinted or reproduced or utilised in any form or by any electronic, mechanical, or other means, now known or hereafter invented, including photocopying and recording, or in any information storage or retrieval system, without permission in writing from the publishers.

Notice:
Product or corporate names may be trademarks or registered trademarks, and are used only for identification and explanation without intent to infringe.

British Library Cataloguing in Publication Data
A catalogue record for this book is available from the British Library

ISBN: 978-1-84872-168-5 (Set)
ISBN: 978-1-138-96467-9 (pbk)
ISBN: 978-1-84872-240-8 (hbk) (Volume 5)

Publisher's Note
The publisher has gone to great lengths to ensure the quality of this book but points out that some imperfections from the original may be apparent.

Disclaimer
The publisher has made every effort to trace copyright holders and would welcome correspondence from those they have been unable to trace.

BILINGUALISM AND LANGUAGE DISABILITY

ASSESSMENT & REMEDIATION

EDITED BY NIKLAS MILLER

CROOM HELM
London & Sydney

COLLEGE-HILL PRESS, INC.
San Diego, CA 92105

© 1984 Niklas Miller
Croom Helm Ltd, Provident House, Burrell Row,
Beckenham, Kent BR3 1AT

Croom Helm Australia Pty. Ltd,
G.P.O. Box 5097, Sydney
NSW 2001, Australia

British Library Cataloguing in Publication Data

Bilingualism and language disability.
1. Bilingualism 2. Children – Language
I. Miller, Niklas
401'09 P115

ISBN 0-7099-1753-8

College-Hill Press, Inc.
4284 41st Street
San Diego, CA 92105

Library of Congress Cataloging in Publication Data
Main entry under title

Bilingualism and language disability

Bibliography: p.
Includes index
1. Bilingualism 2. Language disorders in children
3. Language acquisition. I. Miller, N. (Niklas)
P115.B545 1984 404'.2 84-1929
ISBN 0-933014-26-0

Printed and bound in Great Britain

CONTENTS

LIST OF CONTRIBUTORS

Sam Abudarham, Speech Therapy Department, Birmingham Polytechnic, Birmingham B42 2US, *England*

Eleanor Anderson, Hertfordshire College of Higher Education, Wall Hall, Aldenham, Watford, Herts. WD2 8AT, *England*

Martin Ball, Ysgol Therapi Llafar/School of Speech Therapy, Athrofa Addysg Uwch De Morgannwg/South Glamorgan Institute of Higher Education, Western Avenue, Llandaff, Cardiff CF5 2YB, *Wales*

Sandra Ben-Zeev, Creative Research Associates, 180 N. Michigan Avenue, Chicago, Illinois, *USA*

Eva Gavillán-Torres, Technical Consultant, Suite 405, 3420 16th Street NW, Washington DC 20010, *USA*

Carolyn Kessler, University of Texas at San Antonio, College of Social and Behavioural Sciences, Division of Bicultural-Bilingual Studies, San Antonio, Texas 78285, *USA*

Niklas Miller, Speech Therapy Department, Belfast Hospital for Sick Children, Falls Road, Belfast BT12 6BE, *N. Ireland*

Arturo Tosi, Department of Modern Languages, Oxford Polytechnic, Headington, Oxford OX3 0BP, *England*

ACKNOWLEDGEMENTS

Thanks are due to Croom Helm Publishers who had the foresight in the first place to suggest compiling this volume. Thanks are also due to all the contributors who agreed to apply their knowledge and experience in creating a work in this young field. I would like to thank my colleague Joan Stephenson for some valuable comments regarding style in my own chapters. Any remaining shortcomings in that respect are oversights of my own. My other colleagues are to be thanked for enabling me to pull less than my full weight in the ongoing clinical work during the preparation of the book. Geraldine McKeown and Irene Miller had the unenviable task of typing and retyping scripts, and to them I am gratefully indebted.

Béal Feirste N. Miller

PREFACE

Handicapping conditions do not respect ethnic, geographical, religious or any other boundaries imposed by man. In any population one can expect to find hearing-impaired, blind, cerebral-palsied, mentally-retarded and learning-disabled children. The life-style, social and physical environment and in some cases genetic factors, might predispose certain groups to be more susceptible to particular handicaps. However, to a greater or lesser degree all conditions will be found.

Frequently one of the main casualties in the impairment of normal development that may accompany many of these disabilities is the acquisition of language and its exploitation in both the social and cognitive growth of the child. Over the past two or three decades significant advances have been made in the ability to detect and describe communication difficulties in children from a very early age. Parallel progress has been achieved in our ability to prescribe and carry out remedial programmes to maximise the effectiveness of an individual within his communicative environment. The theories, practices, methods and materials from these advances, however, have all been derived from work with monolingual subjects growing up to be members of a monolingual society.

The twentieth century has witnessed movements of population, from political, economic and other causes, on an unprecedented scale. One consequence of this has been the creation of sizeable bilingual communities throughout the world. Early (and not entirely dispersed) attitudes towards the language development of people within these communities were that eventually they should or would become monolingual, monocultural members of the 'host' society. This is the so-called 'melting-pot' theory. Alternative views have to some extent brought about the reversal of this trend and stressed contributions to the richness of a society that cultural and language pluralism can bring. But the attaining of such pluralistic ideals remains still very much in its infancy. Returning to the position of those handicapped persons who can be expected to be found amongst any bilingual community within a larger predominantly monolingually-oriented society, this recognition of their rights to language and cultural choice has certain implications for effective habilitation of them into the wider non-handicapped population.

Assessment methods and materials have mostly been standardised on a monocultural, monolingual population. The validity of the application of such measures even to other subcultures within a monolingual society is questionable, let alone their accuracy when used with children of markedly different cultural and linguistic backgrounds. This similarly applies to the creation and execution of remedial efforts in helping the handicapped child realise his true potential. The melting-pot approach to development laid any language or other problems fairly and squarely with the 'immigrant' or 'bilingual' and viewed difficulties as arising from their attempts to become or to be made effective monolingual speakers. The pluralistic approach has to respect the diversity that exists and to create and adapt materials for assessment and remediation that are going to be sensitive to these overall societal aims. The problem is no longer to make the subject fit the materials and imposed circumstances, but to make the theories and materials fit the subjects.

Endeavours in this direction, especially in the field of language development of the handicapped child, have only really taken on an air of seriousness and urgency during the past two decades. The area of study is still, particularly in Europe, characterised by disparate efforts, controversy and a lack of overall cohesion and direction in what is required to fulfil the aims and obligations of a pluralist society to the individuals within it. This book has a threefold aim. The first aim is to serve as an introduction to the field of bilingual studies, and the issues in that discipline, for those who have had no previous contact with bilingualism, but who by choice or force of clinical circumstances are obliged to inform themselves about it. Secondly, it is hoped that it offers knowledge and practical directions which will be of assistance to people who are charged with the care of handicapped children from a bilingual-bicultural background. Thirdly, by showing up the gaps in our understanding and elucidating on issues to which answers need to be found, it is also intended as a contribution to the crystallisation of ideas and aims in the sphere of study under discussion.

Bilingualism is both a societal and an individual phenomenon, and the nature of bilingualism is a product of the interaction of variables at these two levels. An appreciation of the linguistic, cognitive and social development of the individual within a bilingual community must commence with an appreciation of the forces that influence that development within any given community. It is against such a background that any diagnostic measures will have to be devised and interpreted, and it is to the demands of this background that management plans will need to be tuned. Chapter 1 attempts to set the scene in this respect. Chapter 2 relates more specifically to language development. An understanding of what constitutes non-normal development will only follow the recognition of normal patterns and it is to this end that such a chapter is included. The third chapter deals with the cognitive aspects of the growth of the individual within the bilingual community. In the past arguments have been waged between those who see a direct causal link between bilingualism and developmental retardation and those who would claim positive benefits from being bilingual. The actual state of affairs is somewhat more complex than one of simple cause and effect and Chapter 3, as well as dispelling earlier myths about the consequences from bilingualism for cognition, aims to elaborate on the true nature of the interrelationship of the two. Chapter 4 works towards an analysis of which language difficulties of bilingual children are more imagined and which ones are more real; which ones are merely reflections of 'problems' faced by any child, mono- or bilingual, in learning to communicate, and which ones might be attributable to the bilingual status itself. Within the latter category a division is discerned between those problems that derive from external circumstances and those that might arise from the individual's internal state.

An awareness of the difficulties posed by cross-cultural assessment is not new. Chapters 5 to 8 review briefly past thoughts and controversies in this area, offer suggestions for current practice and mark out the directions in which scholarship needs to progress to attain maximum fairness and efficiency.

The last three chapters deal with the problems for the monolingual remediator with monolingual materials in the management of the potentially bilingual child diagnosed as having (first)-language acquisition difficulties. Chapter 9 addresses the problems and pitfalls in case-history compilation in cross-cultural settings, while Chapter 10 outlines the basis for remediation and offers practical advice on problems of programme implementation and personnel training. Chapter 11 is included to emphasise the difference between management for children who have only a second-language learning difficulty and those who have problems in learning any language at all. The book is directed chiefly at the management of the latter. It is also, though, included as it is contended that in some cases first- and second-language remediation can complement each other, and practitioners can learn by viewing the solutions that have been arrived at in the respective fields to problems and controversies that have arisen.

The following chapters will probably not answer all the questions that we would wish to find solutions for, in order to carry out effectively our clinical and pedagogical work. Many of the chapters conclude with pleas for further research, further investment in this field of study and the direction of resources and personnel to achieve this. Final answers (if there are any) will only be reached when this has come about. It is hoped that this book, as well as offering suggestions for interim solutions by at least pinpointing the right questions, has also signposted the road to the right answers. The reader must remain aware that answers to the problems posed in handicap and bilingualism will not arise independently of change and answers in society at large.

Part 1

WHAT IS BILINGUALISM?

1 LANGUAGE USE IN BILINGUAL COMMUNITIES

Niklas Miller

Language scholarship entered the second half of the twentieth century still largely under the influence of the attitudes of the nineteenth. The predominant view saw languages describable in terms of one grammar, the correct one, more often than not based on the written texts of classical authors, rather than the spoken language of people at large. Attitudes to foreign languages reflected very much the European missionary and civilising obsessions that saw fit to wipe out or suppress the native languages of the Americas, Africa and Asia, not to mention those of their home continent. Witness the English campaign against Welsh, Irish and Scots Gaelic or Bismarck's attempt to eradicate Polish from Prussian territory. Feelings towards bilinguals (other than maybe between two of the 'prestigious' European languages) were also much coloured by the same obsessions. To speak an inferior language was a sign of inferiority and uneducatedness and bilingualism was seen as a transitional stage on the way to civilisation. All the negative attitudes that were directed at the supposedly inferior cultures and peoples also became attached to bilinguals and bilingualism. Other handicaps were claimed to be associated with bilingualism, including left-handedness, stuttering, mental retardation and schizophrenia. Henss, quoted by Weinreich (1963, p. 119), in addition to these warned that a bilingual child 'begins to brood over its own peculiarities . . . it becomes subject to an inner split'. Where bilingualism was tolerated it was usually expected to be the equal and native-like control of two languages. Linguists and psychologists with their academic directions were also not unresponsible for the delayed recognition of the true nature of bilingualism. The dichotomy between language as a body of rules versus the actual realisation of these rules (de Saussures' *langue* and *parole* and Chomsky's competence and performance) led mainstream linguistics to be centred on abstract aspects of language rather than live usage.

Psychologists, when they did study bilingualism, saw bilinguals simply as those with two languages without attention to their use and functions. Work on the representation of the bilingual's languages within the brain and possible neurophysiological correlates of switching from one language to another was conducted without reference to why or when they might switch. However, with the growth of anthropology, sociolinguistics, social psychology and other fields over the past twenty years and a reawakening to cultural relativism and pluralistic thinking, a more accurate view of bilingualism has emerged. The following offers an overview of what is involved in describing bilingualism and bilinguals.

Describing Bilingual Communities

Bilingual communities may be described along several dimensions. It is important, however, in discussing these to bear in mind that the dimensions are not labels for immutable opposites, for example stable at one pole and unstable at the other pole, but are continua where any given community might be characterised by its relative position on the continuum between two extremes. Another point of consideration is that these dimensions do not operate independently, but typically form a complex system of interacting variables. Hence a bilingual community and the individuals in it are not describable in terms of a list of discrete, absolute characteristics, but are a product of how far and in what ways the various positions on the intersecting continua interact. In so far as no two communities are likely to be at exactly the same position on the continua, and variables interact in a different way, if only slightly, from one context to another, it could be said that no two bilingual communities are the same. Furthermore, different communities tend to be characterised by different sets of continua. While a particular dimension or combination of dimensions might be valid for one instance, it will not necessarily hold true for another – be it for another stage in the community's existence, or, as will be seen below, maybe not even for certain subgroups within a larger descriptive unit. A detailed study of a bilingual situation, then, involves the evaluation of the interaction between a host of historical, political, social, psychological and other variables. Fortunately, despite the heterogeneity amongst bilingual societies, for the present purposes of the assessment and remediation of handicapped children from these settings, a description of the minutiae of the variable factors would be unnecessary. However, it is contended that in assessment and therapy attention must be given to the macro- and microsocial aspects of the child's language environment since these have an important bearing on the overall pattern of language use that the child will have been exposed to, on the attitudes to the learning and maintenance of the languages concerned and to the possible educational and remedial provisions available. They will, for instance, amongst other things, have a bearing on whether the child learns the two (or more) languages simultaneously or consecutively; the use to which the languages will be put; whether it is felt that acquiring another language is an advantage – educationally, socially, economically – or an extra burden; the extent of diversity within the community; whether there exist trends amongst different age, economic or social groupings, towards other patterns of usage; and the social and psychological influences that are liable to impinge on language acquisition and use.

Macrosociolinguistic Variables in Language Usage

This discussion covers variables that will be relevant for the clinician and teacher, but does not deal with all possible dimensions. For an elaboration of these points readers are referred to Giles (ed.) (1977), Anderson (1979), Fishman (1980) and Hudson (1980) on whose works the following to some extent relies.

One broad category of features are the demographic ones. These cover several interdependent continua including whether the bilingual population is an immigrant or indigenous one; of recent origin or long-standing; real and relative numbers of minority-language speakers in relation to majority language; distribution of bilinguals within the wider community, both in terms of density of settlement and rural compared with urban location, with the latter division being closely linked with social factors, discussed below; existence of different bilingual groupings rather than one homogeneous group; and whether these groupings are within a predominantly monolingual society or one accepted as bi- or multilingual and multicultural. Within this last category one could contrast between countries such as Australia, Britain and Germany, where dominant attitudes and institutions are directed towards one language and culture, despite the presence of sizeable bilingual communities, and on the other hand Belgium, Canada and Ireland, where there is legislative recognition of certain rights of coexisting languages and cultures. However, one must also examine the contrast between the constitutionally envisaged ideal and actual practice. This distinction obviously has implications for the maintenance of language use and the permitted scope of educational planning.

Further demographic features include whether the bilingual community is increasing in number – maybe from the continued influx of new immigrants, typical of many European countries, where immigration laws permit, or from urbanisation trends, common in many African states – or decreasing in number. Decrease might result from forced or voluntary emigration or strong intra- or extragroup pressures towards assimilation with the surrounding monolingual community.

Where the bilingual individuals are an isolated family or a small and loosely-knit community of relatively recent arrival in a monolingual community, the likelihood is of a home/non-home split in language usage. Family and home affairs will probably be the only domains of minority-language use, the bilinguals having to use the majority language for all out-of-home purposes. Pressures to become monolingual, especially from peer group, educational and job market directions, will be strong, and while the people may not be actively discriminated against on account of their language, in so far as the majority community is unlikely to make any provision for maintenance of the minority language and because it would fulfil no functions outside the family, this process is liable to proceed unhindered. In time bilinguals here may become passive bilinguals, able to use their original language if needs be, but disinclined to do so. Alternatively those family members who have least motivation to learn the new language, usually those who stay at home, who tend to be elderly people and women, may preserve their old language most, while the others use it only when talking to, or in the presence of, these persons. Mercer, Mercer and Mears (1979) reported just this from interviews with some Gujarati-English bilingual teenagers in Leicester, and Gal (1979), recording processes of change in language choice in Oberwart, noted a similar phenomenon, where some sections of the population are shifting from being Hungarian-German bilinguals to monolingual German-speakers. As it becomes less and less meaningful, culturally, linguistically and pragmatically, for a group or individual to be bilingual, the chance of passing on the skill to succeeding generations diminishes. Thus it is not uncommon to find the first-generation immigrant family most fluent in the minority language, with majority-language knowledge restricted to comprehension and expression necessary for day-to-day survival in the community, typically amounting to a comprehension better than expression; their second-generation children move towards the opposite of this, with minority-language skills restricted to home matters and interpreting for their parents, while they in turn may be reluctant to encourage, or even actively discourage, their own children from using the minority language. Clearly this is not the only picture and different patterns of immigration, settlement and role access will produce other patterns of language-learning and use. More discussion of this matter is given later in this chapter and in Chapter 2.

At the opposite end of the immigrant number and density continua are those areas where there are recognisable concentrations of speakers of the same minority language. Such situations are generally marked by a longer history of immigration, a degree of intragroup support for maintenance of the minority culture and/or language, including through social networks, cultural and religious bodies, ethnic schools (frequently attended in addition to monolingual majority culture education) and a measure of economic independence, in that local stores, service trades and recreational centres might have developed, run by the ethnic minority members for their own community. Also there may be a feeling of contrast with the majority community and a desire to uphold these differences, even though some of the features that initially set the two communities apart might be lost over time.

In these contexts it is quite feasible for some ethnic minority persons to exist without ever actively using the majority language. Their only contact may be through the electronic media, street signs and advertisements. Others may have a limited spoken command sufficient to order goods from a wholesaler, deal with majority-community customers, make enquiries at local and national administrative departments and similar well-defined transactions. In some countries practical provision for schooling in the community language is made. This may vary between, for example, Belgium and Switzerland, where there is opportunity for pursuing studies even to tertiary level in the language of one's choice, and other countries which enable students to attend all or some classes until the end of secondary or primary education in the language they choose. Other countries make no concessions and may even discriminate against all but one favoured language, such as in Britain or New Zealand. The types and nature of bilingual education are discussed in Chapter 11. How far these various provisions and other institutional supports with which they are frequently associated are practically realised and how far they remain purely notional or semi-effective depends on many other community characteristics apart from demographic, including social, economic and political factors.

The possibility for people to commence or carry out all their education in their 'own' language is frequently only one aspect of support or guarantee which a language might be afforded in the legislation or constitution of a society. There may exist articles giving language certain air-time on radio and television, support to publications in those languages, recognition of their status in legal, trade and governmental dealings. The contexts for acquisition and use of languages will naturally be different in those societies where there is institutional support, where pluralism is tolerated, preserved or even encouraged, from those where it is not tolerated or unintentionally, or intentionally, counteracted.

Not all bilingual groups, of course, result from recent immigration. Many are remnants of previously more widespread communities which may have been powerful monolingual cultures in their own right, but have been subjected, divided, redistributed by the redrawing of frontiers, or in countless other ways depleted and obliged to acquire another language to assure their survival. This is true of many American Indian languages or the Celtic languages of Europe. In these cases, as with many immigrant centres, the bilingual speakers may in fact constitute a majority of the inhabitants in a region and have created or maintained a degree of linguistic and cultural life independent of the wider national situation. Quebec and some areas in Belgium (Baetens-Beardsmore, 1980) represent examples of this. The fact that bilingual speakers exist, however, indicates that for certain purposes it is necessary to speak both languages, and that more power, prestige or usefulness may be attached to one language, emphasising how status and support factors are as important as demographic factors in determining language maintenance and choice.

Relative status accorded to one language over another is usually the consequence of a complex interaction of historical and social factors, in the broadest sense, covering religious, cultural, economic and demographic areas. Status here has nothing to do with any inherent property of a language quantifiable in any linguistic sense independent of the social factors. Certain languages may be less adapted to particular functions, such as for use in disseminating information on scientific, musicological or legal matters. However, this will be only secondary to the social functions or status ascribed to them since one of the inherent properties of natural languages is their adaptability. In the Middle Ages it was claimed that the various living languages of Europe would not be able to replace Latin as a medium for serious philosophical or technical discourse, yet in the twentieth century the same claim, in turn, is being made for English, French, German, etc., over other languages. Likewise statements abound claiming that non-standard varieties of languages are incapable of serving other than menial duties, forgetting that today's local vernacular is often tomorrow's standard language.

One almost universally occurring feature in the relationships between languages in contact is the dominant/non-dominant dichotomy. As intimated above, this is a reflection of other broad social circumstances rather than anything emanating directly from any formal qualities of the languages involved. These social circumstances centre round the control of power within the community, whether this be through control of economic, educational, administrational or other resources. In so far as the speakers of one language are in control of these resources, a command of that language will be a prerequisite in gaining access to them and to the power which that access carries. The converse is that lack of the necessary language skills will be a further obstacle to benefitting from the advantages that being party to the power and control sources lends.

One type of dominant/non-dominant language community was described by Ferguson (1959), who noted some situations, relatively stable, where in addition to the primary dialects of a language (including possible regional standards) there was 'a very divergent highly codified . . . superposed variety'. This superposed variety, which he termed the high (H) variety in contrast to the vernacular, low (L) variety, is not used by any members of the community in ordinary conversation and is acquired largely through formal education. It is used in written documents, government, academic, legal and other formal contexts. He labelled such communities diglossic, and cited as examples Greek with its H *katharévusa* and L *dhimotikí*, classical (H) and colloquial (L) Arabic and so on. H is always seen as a prestige variety and some speakers maintain they have no knowledge of L, that H is the 'true' language and L only a debased, corrupt form. The grammar of H is usually more formalised than L and contains more obligatorily marked categories, morpheme-alternants and less symmetrical paradigms (e.g. for number or tense marking). Since the introduction of the term there has been an extension of the types of community H covers. Ferguson originally covered only situations in which H and L were different varieties of the same language, but Fishman (see Fishman, 1980) includes any society in which two or more (hence one could have triglossia) varieties are used under distinct circumstances. It is also used to describe speech communities where H and L are different languages – e.g. English and Filipino as H and Tagalog as L in the Philippines or Spanish H and Guarani L in Paraguay. The essential factor is that access to higher institutions and roles is only granted with use of H, and adherence to H cultural values. The cultural correlate of diglossia has been called diethnia.

The extreme of domination is represented in situations where there is active suppression of a language, or situations which are tantamount to suppression, when no recognition or support is given to a language, either in the schools, the media, or anywhere else. Most European countries until the last decade fell into this latter category, and still have in their general dealings with minority languages the legacy of those attitudes. It is also typical of areas where immigration has not been previously experienced and where numbers are too small to create or uphold the infrastructure for alternative sources of power and control.

The same holds true in Ireland which is nominally a bilingual country, but genuine bilingual usage is restricted to sparsely populated counties away from the main centres of commerce, higher education and national government. Thus for the majority of the people English is preferable to Irish, and to succeed in skilled employment or the business world, English is required. Canada serves as a similar example, where the equality of English and French is legally guaranteed, yet because of the power structure of the country overall, any bilinguals leaving Quebec or the other French-speaking localities will be at a disadvantage. Such a state of affairs has considerable bearing on the motivation to acquire languages and attitudes to their usage. The effects on the actual learning processes involved are discussed in the next chapter, and the implication for cognitive development in Chapter 3.

Until now variation in language use has been spoken of in terms that relate to general macrosociolinguistic trends within or between communities. These, however, are not the only source of variation and are complemented by a network of interacting factors which operate at a microsociolinguistic level influencing variety from individual to individual and from one context of interaction to another.

Microsociolinguistic Variables in Language Usage

As with the discussion of the macrolevel factors influencing synchronic and diachronic variation, the detailing of factors at the microlevel is a discussion of a complex of largely mutually interdependent continua. Hence to separate one from the other is for explicatory purposes only and should not be taken to imply that for any one speaker or group of speakers a given variable is an independently isolatable or existing dimension. Further, while variation is inherent in all language systems, and while it might be possible to enumerate the various dimensions along which this might range, it cannot be assumed that each community will attach the same social significance to the dimensions nor that there is cross-cultural consistency in the nature of the relationship of one continuum to another. Thus while two communities might display patterns of language variation associated with the interaction of the relative ages of interlocutors and topic of conversation, the salience of either and the degree and ways in which they interact will probably be different. This underlines the need to treat each bilingual community individually and not interpret activities of one in terms formulated for another. Another vital aspect is the role of the individual speaker.

Linguists, social anthropologists and the like may make assertions about social and psychological factors and their linguistic correlates, general patterns of usage or whatever, but in the final analysis the individual is not bound to abide by these abstracted 'rules'. In fact it is through the position an individual assumes regarding conformity to any of the conventions implicitly or explicitly recognised by a community that he defines his attitude to an interlocutor or group. This element of variation has been emphasised by Bourhis (1979, p. 119), who stated 'the assumption must be that a speaker's behaviour is never completely determined by social norms and rules within a situation, nor by the effects of sociostructural factors in society. In each instance, individuals' needs, motives, perceptions and attributions must play some part in determining the speech strategy finally encoded or decoded . . .' Le Page (1975) and Halliday (1978) have expressed the same view.

A further vital feature of language variation is its probabilistic, relative, rather than absolute nature. A speaker does not utilise either language or dialect A or language or dialect B in the sense of switching between two extremes, as was the view earlier held in bilingualism. Rather, according to what factors are in operation during an act of communication and according to the attitude a speaker chooses to adopt to those factors, the person's speech will more likely *approximate* to a particular end of a continuum language A → language B, rather than be *exclusively* A or B. Thus a change that is considered by both speaker and listener to be from an informal to formal variety, in monolingual situations, or language A to B in a bilingual setting, need not imply change across all levels of language – phonology, syntax, semantics. It may involve variation in only one or a handful of features. The New York postvocalic /r/ (Labov, 1970), the realisation of the verb participle -ing as /ɪn/ v. /ɪng/ (Trudgill, 1974a) and the presence or not of initial /h/ would be examples of phonological shift markers. In the area of syntax the change might be an increase in the proportion of more complex structures (subordinate clauses, passives, etc.) or expanded rather than elliptical utterances. In lexical choice, a shift in variety might involve the preference for a certain group of words over another, e.g. stomach ache v. abdominal pain, says his t's and k's v. alveolar plosives are realised as velars.

The same holds true for changes in variety in bilingual usage. What an objective, independent observer notes as only an increase in the proportion of lexical items from language B occurring in a stretch of apparently (e.g. phonologically and syntactically) language A utterances, may be perceived by the speaker/listeners involved as the change from one language to another required by the shift in the social or psychological tenor of their exchange. The perceived change might be manifested in an increase in the use of syntactic structures from language B, or the stretches of alternation between A and B contain longer stretches of the one or other language. This has strong implications in assessment and remediation and is a point taken up below.

Statistical methods have been adopted to describe this type of variation. Labov (1970) in his New York studies was the first to use them extensively. Milroy (1980) has employed other statistical techniques in the analysis of language variation and the correlation with social networks. Le Page (see McEntegart and Le Page, 1982) has also attempted to exploit statistical means in describing bidialectal/bilingual variation in Belize and St Lucia. Using this approach, statements on usage become a matter of predicting the statistical probability with which a feature is likely to occur in or be associated with a particular context. Switches from one variety to another are not seen as absolute switches but in terms of an increase or decrease in the probability of appearance of a specified set of features.

This apparent 'confusing' of languages has in the past been one source of prejudice against bilinguals and a factor which has led to misinterpretation of their language use and language competence. It has been a cause for some people to claim that in trying to acquire two languages, bilinguals master neither, and that they debase the languages they speak. Accepting the mixing and switching between languages as the abnormal rather than the normal, psychologists, teachers, linguists and others have acquired an erroneous impression of what could or should be expected regarding the mastery of two languages in bilinguals.

Bilingualism is comparatively rarely the compartmentalisation of one language from the other. More commonly exchanges between bilinguals, and to a degree between bilingual and monolingual speakers, are typified by utterances that are not analysable by reference to a grammar of either the one or the other language which the person is said to speak. Rather from the grammatical, analytical standpoint, utterances will contain features of both languages, and samples of, in monolingual speakers' terms, 'pure' English or Spanish or Hindi will be restricted to well-defined contexts. This is not to say that the bilingual speakers would not on occasions feel they are using a 'pure' variety of a particular language, even though it would not fulfil a monolingual listener's criteria for such a label. This phenomenon of sometimes rapid, sometimes sporadic alternation between apparently Spanish and apparently English, or whatever languages are at the time in question, is termed code-switching. When the two languages are apparently constantly intermingled it is termed code-mixing. Both are typical of bilingual situations (see Parkin, 1977, and Dulay, Hernández-Chávez and Burt, 1978).

It is time to examine some of the influences on language usage that bring about or are parallel to the shifts in language. The factors mentioned below do not by any means exhaust all the possible correlations of social, psychological and linguistic change, not even for one speech community. The number of social and psychological settings one wished to study and the depth of detail one was aiming at would determine just how many factors one would take into account. The features covered here are chosen to give a representative rather than complete picture of how particular influences can interact, and to include ones which have a fair degree of cross-cultural similarity in occurrence and relevance for the present clinical assessment purposes.

Three broad areas of influence within which language variation has been studied are the effects related to the persons involved, the setting/place of their interaction and the topic under discussion. Usage for any one occasion will be a product not only of the interaction between these three variables, but also of variables within each category, and between them and the macrosociolinguistic factors enumerated above.

Factors related to the persons involved may include age, sex, ethnic group, class/caste, geographical provenance (region; rural v. urban; inner city v. suburban), relative role status, in-group/out-group member, and overriding all of these, the interlocutors' willingness to comply with or deny the linguistic conventions that would normally operate in the presence of any of these factors.

Age-related speech styles are associated either with the age of the listener or of the speaker. Young children do not use the same range of syntactic structures and lexicon as their teenage siblings who in turn use different styles to their parents and grandparents. Jahangiri and Hudson (1982) speculate on some of the possible forces operating to create such variation. Differences according to the age of the interlocutor include varieties spoken when addressing children or babies, those used when speaking to one's peers and for talking with older persons. Clearly these factors would seldom operate in isolation and other personal and situational determinants (see below) interact closely with them. In bilingual communities the switch in varieties according to age can involve switches in language. The examples already quoted from Gal (1979) and Mercer *et al.* (1979) illustrate this.

Differences in speech related to the sexes of the speakers also fall into two types. First are quantitative variations along various continua. One widely reported example of this is the tendency of women to use a higher percentage of features towards the prestige end of the vernacular-prestige continuum when compared with their age, class and educationally matched male counterparts. Labov (1970) found this in New York and more recently the same trends have been described by Milroy (1980) in Belfast and Jahangiri and Hudson (1982) in Teheran. There is also a tendency for women to retain more conservative forms and men to be innovative, though as prestige and conservative features are often closely associated it is not always clear whether this represents a separate phenomenon (cf. Trudgill, 1974, p. 90).

The second class of variation is qualitative. In British English, qualitative differences between male-male and male-female conversation, where the feature 'female' is a salient factor, might include what could be loosely labelled 'more polite speech'. Certain lexical items are favoured, the tone and rate of speech are modified, and the males may approximate more to the prestige-oriented female forms. However, many speech communities exist where alternative syntactic, morphological or phonological markers are obligatory. Trudgill (1974) gives the example of the Gros Ventre Amercian Indian speakers where palatalised dental stops in men's speech correspond to the women's palatalised velar stops; or Darkhat Mongolian where men and women use different vowel series. He also quotes the celebrated example of the Carib Indians where the men and women spoke such divergent versions of the language that the first Europeans to encounter them thought they were speaking different languages.

The race of the interlocutor may exert an influence on the choice of language. This may result from affective factors associated with particular ethnic groups or subgroups (prejudice, solidarity, suspicion, etc.) or the status (see immediately following) of certain races within a society. Irrespective of these factors, usage may be determined by the fact that certain groups are known not to be bilingual and hence only one particular language may be spoken to them – e.g. Gujarati-speakers in England might communicate with other Indian subcontinent language speakers in Hindi or English. Amongst the English and West Indians, Hindi is unknown, hence with them English would be the language of choice.

Status factors represent a strong source of influence on language choice. By status is meant a person's standing in relation to others and in the eyes of others. There is no one constant dimension to status since each group and subgroup applies its own criteria in assigning importance to personal roles. Hence the value system used to judge relative status in one community cannot be taken as valid for another, nor can it be assumed that each person within a community necessarily shares the same set of criteria. Witness, for instance, the common differences that exist towards (establishment) law enforcers or politicians and the varying status of elders, aunts, uncles, mothers and elder siblings within a family grouping; or in the one individual, the changes in the status ascribed to teachers between primary school, secondary school and later as a parent, not to mention cross-culturally the different attitudes to the 'disciplined' teachers in the ethnic school compared with the 'western' teachers and their perceived poor control (cf. Noble and Ryan, 1979 and Triseliotis, 1976). People who feel they are disadvantaged by a class/caste system may demonstrate their disapproval, amongst other ways, through non- or only partial compliance to the linguistic conventions generally correlating with class variations.

Further, a person's status relative to another can alter according to the role they are performing – e.g. father to child as moral preacher and as playmate; or according to the varying role factors that become the focus of attention at various stages of a transaction – e.g. a black, male parent talking to a younger, white female teacher focusing initially on her higher status as a teacher and the fact that she is a female, but later changing the speech style as whiteness and youth (less experienced) become more salient features.

The interaction between language use and social structure is by no means straightforward, and it is impossible to do justice to it in this chapter. Halliday (1978) has discussed the relationship between the two. A person's command of intra- or interlanguage variations is seen as a function of their positions and allegiances within a social stratificational matrix. However, their command of language varieties is also influenced by the range of roles to which they have access, which is a function of this same position within the social hierarchy. In this way, language, as well as being a product of these social forces, is also a force in itself that under certain circumstances can facilitate access to new social positions. As Halliday (1978, p. 186) points out, 'In a typical hierarchical structure, dialect becomes the means by which a member gains, or is denied, access to certain registers', demonstrating that (p. 183) 'the relation of language to the social system is not simply one of expression but a more complex natural dialectic in which language actively symbolises the social system, thus creating as well as being created by it'.

Attitudes to acquisition and usage of particular languages or varieties can be greatly influenced by the status and potential power that is invested in a person who has command of them. As well as influencing acquisition, the status factor can also result in some families or groups neglecting or abandoning languages which they view as having low status. Attention is drawn in this connection to the discussion of semi-lingualism in Chapters 2, 4 and 11.

Different communities utilise varying ways of signalling relative status in language. In British English, speakers select phonological and lexicogrammatical positions on the continua between the local vernaculars and the assumed elite standard forms. Status also affects paralinguistic features such as body posture and distance, physical and eye contact, who is allowed to interrupt or question whom, who is permitted to change topic or break off the transaction. Cross-cultural variation clearly exists in these aspects, and the way in which this can lead to misunderstandings is elaborated upon on pages 92-3, 133, 137.

Remaining with strictly linguistic markers, some languages – e.g. Japanese – maintain a whole system of honorifics for use with interlocutors of different status. In Korean (Trudgill, 1974), degrees of status can produce considerable grammatical and lexical variation. There are six obligatory verb suffixes to choose between in marking relative status. In the languages of India different language styles are associated with the different castes.

In bilingual communities these variations may be reflected not only in intralanguage alternations, but also in interlanguage switching. The diglossic situations described above provide prime examples of where this occurs.

All these choices are subject to the proviso that a choice does in fact exist (see the Hindi-English choice above), and that the speaker(s) are willing to acknowledge the recognised conventions. Declining to adhere to the linguistic 'laws' of a situation can be as potent a way of demonstrating rejection of a person and/or their values, as acknowledgement and sharing markers can be a strong signal of solidarity. It is in this way that language (even down to the use of particular vowel forms or lexical items) can become a focus of ethnic identity or conflict and a method of enforcing in-group and out-group membership – cf. Parkin (1977) and Russell (1982), or the problems of credibility and acceptance in England for non-standard language-speakers in positions where standard speakers feel they themselves hold a monopoly.

Status and other personal attributes do not operate as independent factors and the effects of relative status may be modified in the light of further forces. One such area is the effect of setting. One may distinguish between physical and symbolic setting. Physical setting refers to the actual place in which a transaction takes place – clinic, school (ethnic v. state), stadium, home, place of worship and so on. In bilingual communities certain languages may be conventionally associated with particular settings. In some cases the use of some languages may even be decreed or forbidden by legislation – e.g. in schools, court or the media. The pattern of settlement and extent of minority community economic and educational infrastructure clearly will have a bearing on the measure of physical settings in which one or other or both of a person's languages are spoken.

It may be possible for some ethnic minority members to avoid ever speaking the dominant language if their local stores, service industries and entertainments are run by people from their own community. What little active knowledge of the dominant language they do possess may be limited to well-defined transactions such as purchasing wholesale goods, settling gas and electricity bills or exchanging the time of day. Children may commence school with only a passive knowledge of English from watching TV or hearing others in their environment speaking it to one another but not to the child himself.

A full appreciation of the relevance of a group's or individual's languages and their competence in them must include an appraisal of the pattern of usage of those languages according to place. A child is unlikely to be familiar with the L2 lexical and grammatical items for fields he has had only L1 contact with. Similarly, because a child is able to talk about some cartoons and gangster programmes on TV and some aspects of playground and street interaction, it does not imply that he would cope with the language required in the classroom or clinic.

Symbolic setting refers to the event taking place in a setting, whatever its physical characteristics. Thus, for example, a rock concert in church, a bingo session at school or a prayer meeting at work may reverse the normal pattern of usage for those physical settings.

The topic of conversation serves as another variable in language choice. Talk amongst bilinguals about L1 cultural matters – home, religion, relations, etc. – is more likely to involve L1 even if the setting is not directly related to that topic. Conversely discussion related to L2 cultural matters – e.g. work, state education, rock music, administrative affairs – will more likely be conducted in that language.

It should be stressed again here, that while interaction is between bilinguals, choice of L1 or L2 is not to be taken as 'pure' L1 or L2, but only to the degree to which the interlocutors feel it is necessary to signal Englishness or Punjabiness.

Another form of topic-based alternation is when there occurs a metaphorical switch within an exchange. Here the switch derives not so much from the subject or the topic but from the tenor of the conversation. Monolinguals will be familiar with changes in dialect, especially in joke or storytelling, to depict the urban sophisticate, the rural numbskull, the trendy teenager, or whatever. They will also be familiar with linguistic changes used to signal humorousness, sarcasm, nostalgia or anger. Such variation exists in the language of bilinguals also, with the added factor that it may encompass a switch from one language to another. Indeed in many communities this ability to exploit the subtleties or powers of association of language in narration and oration may be a prized skill.

Further influences on language choice broadly connected with topic include the reasons for, or purpose of, an exchange. Language may vary according to whether the speaker's purpose is narrative, didactic, interrogatory, suppliant or emphatic. In these circumstances the choice of language may signal or underline the basic intention. Asides and additives form another source of switching. Referrals back in a conversation to a prior topic, or insertion of extraneous pieces of information, or anecdotes, reporting exchanges transacted in another language, all might result in code-switching.

At the microsociolinguistic level, language choice then will be a product of the interaction between the broad categories of person, place and topic and the subsidiary factors assumed under these headings. They may dictate choice for long stretches of discourse, or they may bring about rapid shifts at analytically more local levels. This all assumes that a choice is more than just notionally present and that the individual elects to accept that choice.

To close, a slightly closer look will be taken at examples to examine the practical application of the general influences covered above and to summarise the type of analysis needed by a clinician or teacher in the appreciation of the sociolinguistic background which will be shaping a child's language usage.

Leicester, England, has a population, excluding the extensive suburbs, of approximately 300,000 of whom an estimated 17 per cent (Wilding, 1981) are of Indian subcontinent extraction. As this population is concentrated in only certain parts of the city, this means that particular districts have high (> 50 per cent) ratios of Indian subcontinent people to English ancestry inhabitants. In addition to them there are also sizeable Caribbean, African and Chinese communities who, as with the Indians, have arrived in the city over the past twenty years. Eastern, Central and Southern Europeans constitute longer-established groups of non-English speakers.

Focusing on the Indian subcontinent community, it will be seen that it is clearly not a homogeneous group. By far the largest language communities are Gujarati- and Punjabi-speakers, but Urdu, Hindi and other languages are also spoken. However, the diversity does not end there, as the Indian Asian population can be further broadly divided into those who have an immediate Indian, predominantly rural origin, an East African, mainly urban origin, but still with some ties to India, and an increasing number who were born in Leicester and consider themselves native English. The language divisions also largely coincide with religious differences – Punjabi-speakers being mainly Sikhs, Gujarati-speakers Hindus, and Urdu-speakers Moslems. Hence there exists a heterogeneous overall community with diverse cultural, linguistic and national affiliations.

Density of settlement has permitted the establishment in certain districts of a considerable economic infrastructure which includes supermarkets, food shops, electrical and other household goods outlets, car dealers, estate agents, restaurants, cinemas and social clubs as well as temples and doctors. Furthermore, while attendance at English-language state schools is compulsory, numerous other-language supplementary schools are run. Although there are some all-Indian workshops and businesses, most adults in employment are obliged to seek jobs in English-owned works. Within these communities it is possible for people to lead their lives without actually ever coming into contact with English-speakers, other than maybe through the electronic media and in a limited number of clearly defined transactional contexts – e.g. buying something not purchasable in a local shop or maintaining machinery at work. This is particularly the case for caretakers of preschool children, and the preschool children themselves.

It is further relevant to consider what English, for those who do speak it, is encountered. The English heard by the school-age population, though not necessarily spoken by them, will be the language of education, most probably from teachers using a local variation of the national standard accent. At school they will also hear from their monolingual English peers the syntax, lexicon and phonology of the dialect of Leicester. English is, however, also used as a *lingua franca* between speakers of Gujarati, Punjabi, Urdu, etc. The usage of English in these cases, especially if it is the English the children have brought from their parents and own community, may, however, be at variance with standard English usage. It might be heavily influenced by the variety of English learned by their parents in India, by English as spoken amongst Asians in East Africa, or by what parents consider as 'English' – being mindful of what has been said above regarding relative switches and real versus imagined usage rather than absolute switches from L1 to L2. English here may be far from standard English and be better characterised with its extensive non-English lexical insertion and syntactic and phonological mixing as an interlanguage between English and the other languages.

Exposure to written English will also be far from standard and not represent any direct link with spoken language. First reading books have a syntax and lexicon of their own, adverts on streets, on TV and the headlines of newspapers also have idiosyncratic grammar. This, of course, is true also for monolingual English children, but they at least will have been exposed to a greater variety of spoken English. Some children will have been introduced to literacy in their L1 at ethnic schools.

Opposed to this will be comparatively broad experience of non-English languages at home and in the community – broad in the sense of locations in which it will have been used and topics covered, but also in the sense that other non-English languages might have been heard. Hindi and to a lesser degree Urdu are used by some to communicate with Asians of another first language, as well as in religious observance. Many of the East African Indians would also have a knowledge of Swahili.

Such information is significant in formulating an overall assessment of a child's communicative competence, not only from the point of view of what languages a child has been exposed to, but also the quantity and quality (social, geographical, topic, setting and 'interlanguage' varieties) of that exposure. Such information is also relevant in disclosing what languages and varieties thereof a child requires in order to function effectively as a member of its community, and in guaging the attitudes of the individual family or wider group to the acquisition and maintenance of the languages available. The evaluation of these attitudes demands attention to wider cultural values and ambitions.

Remaining with the Leicester example, a teacher or clinician seeking details of language use would need to be aware of facts, such as, according to the sample covered by Wilding (1981, p. 43), 95 per cent of parents feel it important for their children to speak Asian languages – for cultural and religious reasons, personal and ethnic identity, and facilitation of links with other Asians in Britain and abroad; or, Wilding (1981, p. 22), that a quarter of the respondents experienced difficulties in using English, and films and reading matter in Asian languages were more popular than English-language ones. This would have to be taken in conjunction with the high expectations of most Asian parents for their children educationally, especially their sons, which to be fully realised would require a good command of English. Similarly, any skilled form of employment would require a sound knowledge of English.

These points regarding ascertainment of the pattern of language development and usage for an individual within a particular community and the meaning of language and influences of their culture and situation that exist for a family is emphasised throughout this book. Mercer *et al.* (1979) in their brief survey cover some of the cultural factors that might be considered in decisions on designing assessment and remediation material, especially the link between ethnic identity and attitudes to maintenance of Indian languages. They also point to the importance of not assuming subgroup homogeneity in ethnic identity and aspirations, and emphasise that self-identity need not necessarily be stable across different social settings involving different participants.

Studies of other specific settings outlining factors operating to determine language choice in bilinguals include Ma and Herasimchuk (1968), Elías-Olivares (1976), MacKinnon (1977) and Parkin (1977), while J. Richards (1972) discusses the effects on learning and variety of different acquisition contexts.

In so far as the same variables can be said to be operating in monolingual settings, studies from language choice and variation in that field can be significant to bilingual studies (Macaulay, 1977; Milroy, 1980; Romaine (ed.), 1982).

Recording Language Usage

Part of the assessment of the bilingual child necessitates establishing a profile of his linguistic usage. As stressed above, a simple statement of 'he speaks A and B, with B the better' is entirely inadequate. It is the acceptance of such shallow views of bilingualism which has been responsible for a great deal of the misleading results of studies with bilinguals. A much more sophisticated approach to language usage in bilingual communities has to be adopted to gain a reliable picture that will provide a valid basis for assessment and possible intervention. The gathering of data for such an analysis is not without its problems, and some of these might be mentioned.

Problems of corpus-gathering are not specific to bilingual situations, and the general difficulties associated with this work have been amply aired elsewhere. Issues involved include the nature of the interactions to be sampled, the settings in which these should take place, the materials and techniques to be employed for input and elicitation of data and methods of recording and annotating respondents' behaviour. Further, issues arise in deciding on methods of describing, formalising and interpreting data, with differences deriving both from the psycholinguistic theoretical position of the analyst and from the purpose of the investigation – whether as part of an academic study or in assessing a child's communicative competence with a view to educational placement and intervention. Bloom and Lahey (1978), Chapman (1981), J. Miller (1981) and Crystal (1982) offer views on data collection and analysis. Ingram (1976), Grunwell (1982) and Ball (this volume) discuss the same issues in connection with phonological assessment.

Bilingual usage has been characterised as varying according to who speaks what language to whom, when, where, how and why. To gain as representative a sample as possible it is necessary to account for as many of these variables as is feasible for a given context. It is not likely that simply taking a single clinic/school and a home-based sample, which might be adequate for monolingual settings, will suffice to capture the full variety of bilingual language interaction.

One approach that has been used to achieve a balanced overview of usage is the questionnaire and diary technique. These will be familiar to linguists and psychologists from child studies, and to clinicians in monitoring and assessing behaviours that do not lend themselves to restricted clinical observation – e.g. stuttering, functional communication of dysphasics, or mentally retarded. With modification these can prove valuable in bilingual assessment.

Questionnaires and diaries have sought to define the interpersonal input to the child – i.e. who speaks what languages to him, and what languages does the child hear in his environment, even though not addressed directly to him; what is the percentage input of the L1 relative to L2; can input for a particular language be correlated with identifiable persons in the child's life (grandparents, playmates, etc.) and does variation correspond to different social domains, e.g. home, school, neighbourhood, religion, employment? These findings have to be set against the more general patterns of usage within the community. Relevant also are the aspirations and allegiances of the group, family or individual and the role which language plays in symbolising or realising these. The pressures exerted by the dominant and minority cultures to use certain languages should also be attended to.

Gal (1979), for her research on language use in Oberwart, questioned informants about the domains of church, health service, work, shopping, school and entertainment as well as interpersonal usage with their kin, neighbours, pals and their general attitudes to German and Hungarian. Other questionnaires devised for research, but which provide a detailed framework for eliciting information on language usage, are the survey booklets (adult and child versions) of the British Linguistic Minorities Project (Saifullah-Khan, 1980) or Wilding (1981).

Redlinger (1977) has designed a language background questionnaire for use with bilingual families to assist in defining a child's linguistic and sociolinguistic milieu. The questionnaire is filled in by the mother or caretaker and permits, on the basis of a twelve-hour working day, the mathematical calculation of mean language input to the child, mean language output and 'background noise' – language spoken by family members in which the child is not immediately involved. Areas of enquiry, similar to the research-oriented batteries, include ratings of usage on a five-point scale (exclusively L1 to exclusively L2) between the child and significant others, between others in the child's presence; in electronic and printed media; in situational contexts (scolding, consoling etc.); and general attitudes to usage.

Questionnaire and self-report procedures have been criticised as unreliable. Teitelbaum (1979) reported the difficulty of young children (kindergarten, first grade) in accurately reporting on language usage, a trend which she found reversed with age. The children in Teitelbaum's survey perhaps demonstrated unreliability due to lack of metalinguistic awareness and difficulties with terms such as 'more' and 'less' However, with older subjects, discrepancies between actual and perceived usage arise from other sources.

It was previously stated that switches between languages are often not complete changes from L1 to L2 but shifts along a continuum between them. The situationally demanded marking of L1-ness or L2-ness may be signalled by the introduction of key L1 or L2 features, while preserving a high degree of other language structure. Thus answers to questionnaires/diaries are more likely to be statements of what people *think* they are or should be talking on any particular occasion. Blom and Gumperz (1972) provide a clear example of this with the

Hemnes, Norway, students who denied they had used standard language forms in their discussion of university matters when home on vacation amongst their native dialect-speaking acquaintances. An independent observer's view of proceedings on purely linguistic (as opposed to social-psychological) grounds is likely to give a different picture to what people say they do, or think they themselves or other groups do, or ought to do. The same holds for monolingual speakers. Speakers of received pronunciation English would vigorously deny they 'drop their aitches' or introduce a connecting /r/ in sequences such a 'draw Ursula his face', or ever split their infinitives.

To enable accurate data collection, the involvement of an outside observer (in so far as this will not disrupt normal usage) or analysis of tape-recorded material may be advisable. This is not to say that the informants' own ideas on what they might be speaking are not relevant. Indeed the discrepancy between what parents or child think they are speaking, and a clinician's or teacher's opinion on the same, might represent one source of language difficulty.

An alternative or supplement to introducing persons or recording equipment into a situation is to use diary records by parents. They can be trained to recognise and record chosen aspects of behaviour, training which has to take place in monolingual situations, too. J. Miller (1981) outlines the carrying out of these procedures.

Questionnaires and diaries do not replace standardised tests and analyses in bilingual settings, but are an imperative adjunct to them. They provide a method of evaluating an individual's attitudes to language use as well as defining those settings to be assessed in gaining a reliable profile of a child's language competence. It is not sufficient to accept one sample of clinic- and of home-based language as giving a full picture without first having ascertained the potential variety within and between settings that a child encounters.

Conclusion

This chapter has aimed to outline the social, psychological and linguistic dimensions that must be involved in any consideration of a bilingual's language background and usage. It has tried to present a model that does not view bilingualism with the prescriptivist, ethnocentric attitudes which typified much of our earlier thoughts on the subject, upholding the primacy of written language, referring to classical sources for arbitration on 'correctness', and which demanded equal command of two languages from bilingual speakers, confused social prejudices with linguistic objectivity, and in obliging (passively or forcibly) a person to ignore their mother tongue denied a whole part of their character and existence. Rather the model favoured, following Gumperz (1964), has been that 'Wherever several dialects or languages appear regularly as weapons of language choice, they form a behavioural whole, regardless of grammatical distinctiveness, and must be considerd constituent varieties of the verbal repertoires.' This consideration demands attention to the broader community or national context within which the bilingual group is set – the demographic, constitutional, historical, social and political relationship of the groupings and the bearing this has on attitudes to acquiring and using different languages; the meaning and roles of the language for and in a community, and the forces of educational and vocational expectations and 'reality' that impinge on language development and usage. It also demands attention to *why*, in everyday usage, a person should speak a particular variety of L1 or L2, *how* he speaks it, *when* and to *whom*. An approach adopting an essentially participant, setting and topic taxonomy of interacting variables was touched upon in analysing the how, when, who and wherefore of language choice, with switching taken not as from 'pure' L1 or L2, but along a sliding scale between them.

The implications for assessment and remediation of these points are clear, and many will be elaborated upon in the following chapters. A bilingual child's communicative competence is a product of the nature of his/her exposure to the languages involved – where (s)he has heard them, who was using them, what they were speaking about at the time, how they were using them and why. The two languages do not develop in a parallel, identical manner, even if the child's underlying cognitive capacity does permit this. From the outset in bilingual communities there is liable to be differentiation of usage between the shades of L1 → L2, and learning this pattern is as much a part of the acquisition process as is the development of phonology and syntax. The pattern of variation is not a static, immutable set of rules, but may change, either alongside developments at a national, community or individually-based level (e.g. when entering school, moving house, gaining a new playmate).

In planning assessment and remediation, the needs of the child should be foremost. Teachers/therapists must be aware of the exposure to language and linguistic attitudes the child has experienced and adjust their aims to provide a level and variety of language(s) development that are going to enable the child to achieve optimum communicative efficiency within its environment. This chapter, it is hoped, has set the contextual scene in preparation for how such a goal might be approached.

2 LANGUAGE ACQUISITION IN BILINGUAL CHILDREN

Carolyn Kessler

Becoming bilingual, whether in infancy or in later childhood, is a formidable task for children. Like monolingual first-language development, the acquisition of two languages essentially evolves out of trying to carry on a conversation with someone, an adult caretaker or another child. These efforts at social interaction strike at the heart of language development from the beginning. Developing the communicative competence to achieve success in conveying and understanding meaning in its many aspects is a time-consuming, highly complex process that reaches far beyond surface assessments of sounds, words and sentences. The process of becoming bilingual is a dynamic one, engaging and challenging children's ability to use two language systems for communication with speakers of differing languages and cultures.

Becoming bilingual is further compounded for children by the timing for the acquisition of two languages. For some children the process begins at or nearly at the onset of language, in infancy, as a result of dual language input from parents or other caretakers. The result is first-language bilingualism (Swain, 1972), a process of simultaneously acquiring two languages. This type of developmental bilingualism is described for the acquisition of two languages before age 3, a somewhat arbitrary point which takes into account that children normally by this age have much of the first language (L1) system. When the process of acquiring another language begins after this point, sequential or successive bilingualism occurs in which one language follows, or is second to, the first in the acquisition order. This defines second-language acquisition for both children and adults. In addressing the issue of second-language (L2) acquisition for children, however, it is helpful to distinguish L2 acquisition in the preschool years from that in the school years when the child is at higher maturational levels and when literacy, reading and writing tasks also become part of the total process of becoming bilingual. In discussing language development processes in bilingual children, these three types of child bilingualism will be considered: (1) simultaneous bilingualism in very young children; (2) sequential bilingualism in preschool children; (3) sequential bilingualism in school-age children below the age of puberty.

Theoretical Framework for Bilingual Language Acquisition

The development of bilingualism is a social process that is, unlike monolingualism, a non-universal achievement and, as such, may develop along a continuum ranging from full proficiency in two languages to a minimal degree of competency in one of the languages. In any case, bilingualism results from efforts to communicate, to take part in that interpersonal, interactive process defined by the social situations in which it occurs. Communication, more precisely, may be viewed as the exchange and negotiation of information between at least two persons through verbal and non-verbal symbols, oral and written or visual modalities as well as production and comprehension processes (Canale, 1983). Information is taken here in its broad sense of consisting of conceptual, sociocultural, affective and other content. Communication as a form of social interaction, following Morrow (1977), necessarily involves a high degree of unpredictability and creativity in both the form and content of the message. It takes place in sociocultural contexts through various types of discourse that place constraints on appropriate language use. Additionally, it occurs under limiting conditions such as those imposed by normal maturational processes in children as well as other psychological or environmental constraints such as fatigue, anxiety, background noise or memory. Of critical importance to understanding the process of becoming bilingual, communication always has a purpose, or function, as that of informing, expressing oneself, persuading, entertaining, establishing social relations. It uses authentic, not contrived language, and is judged successful on the basis of its outcomes.

Communicative Competence

It is against this outline of the nature of communication that we can look more closely at the notion of communicative competence to put the various dimensions of bilingual language acquisition in perspective. Canale and Swain (1980) and Canale (1983) stress that communicative competence is an essential part of actual communication. It refers both to knowledge, what one knows consciously or unconsciously about the language and other aspects of communicative language use, as well as to the skill in how well one can use this knowledge in actual communication. This competence includes, then, both the knowledge and the skill which underlie actual communication in a systematic and necessary way.

This theoretical framework for communicative competence identifies four areas of knowledge and skill. The four components include grammatical or linguistic competence, sociolinguistic competence, discourse competence and strategic competence. To appreciate fully the task of becoming bilingual, either for a child or adult, it is necessary to examine the nature of each of these components, which, taken together, give a reasonably comprehensive view of what is involved in the process of language acquisition.

Grammatical Competence. Also called linguistic competence, this component of communicative competence refers to the mastery of formal features of language, the language code. It includes the ability to recognise at a subconscious level the phonological, syntactic and lexical features of a language and the skill to combine these features in pronunciation, word formation and sentence formation. An understanding of the developmental stages for grammatical competence gives important insights into the nature of child bilingualism.

Sociolinguistic Competence. This component addresses the sociocultural rules of language use which define the appropriate use of language. Appropriateness depends on the social context in which language is used. This requires taking into account the status and roles of the participants in the setting, the purposes of the interaction, the norms or conventions of interaction. It involves knowing what to say in a situation and how to say it or even when to say nothing and remain silent. Sociolinguistic competence includes both appropriateness of meaning and appropriateness of form. As Canale (1983) explains, the former refers to the degree to which the expression of particular language functions, attitudes and ideas is judged to be acceptable for a specific situation. For example, while it is often appropriate for a parent or teacher to say to a young child 'Be quiet' or 'Stop that', it is normally very inappropriate for the child to address such utterances to an adult. Appropriateness of form concerns both verbal and non-verbal forms, the use of appropriate register or style in accompaniment with appropriate gestures, facial expressions, tone of voice, spatial relations and the various other dimensions of rules of kinesics and proxemics (J. Richards, 1981).

Sociolinguistic competence is crucial in interpreting utterances for their social meaning. Although we have no written description of all the rules of sociolinguistic competence governing a language, adult native speakers know these rules and use them to communicate successfully in different situations. For children, this is an intricate developmental process that, like grammatical competence, takes place over time and reflects aspects of normal maturational processes. Although studies of the development of pragmatics, rules for using language appropriately, comprise a growing body of literature (Bates, 1976), little is yet known about the normal developmental paths for this interface between linguistic, cognitive and cultural competence for normal L1 development. Even less is known about that for child bilinguals. Nevertheless, sociolinguistic competence is no less important than grammatical competence.

Discourse Competence. Discourse competence is concerned with the connection of a series of utterances to form a meaningful entity. While discourse competence also applies to written language, for purposes of addressing this component in children, we may think of it in reference to the spoken language. Because of the critical role it plays in language development, an understanding of the nature of conversation, in contrast to other speech events such as lectures, interviews, debates, gives insights into the development of discourse competence.

As Richards and Schmidt (1983) point out, conversation is more than merely the exchange of information. It is a form of interaction in which participants bring to the process shared assumptions and expectations about what conversation is, how it develops, and the types of contributions each participant is expected to make. It is constructed from rules governing the introduction of topics, openings and closings, the pairing of utterances, and turn-taking conventions. Discourse competence utilises both grammatical competence, the knowledge and use of language structures, and sociolinguistic competence, the constraints imposed by particular sociocultural contexts, and, additionally, those rules which provide for an ongoing, developing, related succession of utterances. The connections between a series of utterances that join to make a meaningful whole are achieved through cohesion in form and coherence in meaning.

Cohesion deals with overt markers linking utterances, structures which includes conjunctions, such as *and then* or *meanwhile*, or pronouns referring to previously identified persons or events, such as *he*, *it* or *that (made me happy)*. Coherence, in contrast to cohesion, is often achieved without an overt connection. It is based on general knowledge of the real world and familiarity with specific contexts (Savignon, 1983). Violation of discourse rules is exemplified in the example taken from Widdowson (1978, p. 25):

Speaker A: What did the rain do?
Speaker B: The crops were destroyed by the rain.

Although B's reply conforms to rules of both grammatical and sociolinguistic competence, it does not connect well with A's question, violating a discourse rule governing cohesion.

Like other aspects of communicative competence, the development of discourse competence is a long process for children, taking place over many years.

Strategic Competence. This competence is characterised by the strategies drawn on to compensate for breakdowns in communication resulting from imperfect knowledge of the rules in one or more aspects of communicative competence. Native speakers turn to their strategic competence under conditions of fatigue, memory lapses, distraction, anxiety or some other factor affecting language performance. Strategic competence is also used to achieve certain rhetorical effects such as a change in degree of loudness to get attention or make a point. For second-language learners, Corder (1981) distinguishes two types of strategies: communication strategies and learning strategies. The former are devices used to communicate effectively. Learning strategies are mental processes used to construct the rules of a language. Communicative competence includes the ability to adapt one's strategies to a variety of changing conditions. Paraphrase, repetition, circumlocution, message modification, hesitation, avoidance are all strategies used to meet the demands of ongoing communicative interaction. The coping or survival strategies needed to keep channels of communication open are available to all language users. As Corder (1981) hypothesises, at least some of the strategies utilised in second-language acquisition are substantially the same as those in L1 acquisition. Furthermore, in early stages of L2 development, children may have need for specific strategies, a need which may change as a function of both age and degree of L2 proficiency.

In summary, communicative competence results from a complex interaction of grammatical, sociolinguistic, discourse and strategic competence. The precise nature of this interaction is still very much open to speculation. For the developing bilingual, the acquisition of communicative competence in two languages must further take into account the interaction between two language systems. The notion of universals in each of the communicative competence components as well as that of transfer from one language system to another leave open many questions regarding processes of becoming bilingual for children. A measure of sociolinguistic competence and strategic competence allows a degree of communicative competence even before the acquisition of formal rules of grammatical competence. Universal rules of social interaction and an effort or need to communicate through non-verbal means may serve to get meaning across without the use of language. In whatever complex ways the various components interact, the whole of communicative competence is always something other than the simple sum of all its parts (Savignon, 1983).

Many gaps exist in an understanding of bilingual communicative competence, both in its development and in its functioning when viewed against this theoretical framework which focuses on the interaction of the various components. This outline gives, however, an approach to study the process of becoming bilingual, giving an overview of what it is that bilingual children must acquire. Of critical importance, in addition, is the context of the interaction within which acquisition takes place: the language environment, in particular, the language input, and the individual variables children bring to the situation.

Language Environment

In current second-language acquisition a distinction is hypothesised between language acquisition and language learning (Krashen, 1981, 1982). Language acquisition is a natural, subconscious process that occurs in informal environments when the focus is on communication or meaning. It is through this process that children acquire a first language and through which children become bilingual. Language learning, in contrast, is a conscious process that occurs in formal learning environments, as in certain activities at school, and focuses on language form, grammatical competence. It is viewed as being available to older children, probably around puberty, and adults developing a second language. Of the two processes, language acquisition is central. Language learning simply develops a system to edit language output.

Krashen (1982) further argues that the true causative variables in L2 acquisition derive from the amount of comprehensible language input that the acquirer receives and understands and the strength of the affective filter, the set of affective variables that, taken together, provide the degree to which the learner is open to receive language input.

The most important characteristic of input is that it is comprehensible, that it makes sense. This is often achieved when the person who is providing the input uses a slower rate and clearer articulation, more high-frequency vocabulary, fewer idioms and syntactic simplification with shorter sentences. Caretakers appear to do this intuitively with young children acquiring L1. Sensitive second-language teachers also do it.

Optimal input is interesting and relevant to the acquirer. This, of course, varies with levels of cognitive development and life experiences. Furthermore, input is not grammatically sequenced. Unsequenced, natural input, Krashen hypothesises, will contain such a rich variety of structures that it will meet the child at appropriate developmental needs, providing structures a bit beyond the current level of language competence. Input must also be provided in sufficient quantity to make enough 'just right' input for acquisition processes to take hold. Providing concrete 'here and now' experiences which involve the child contributes to meeting requirements for optimal input.

The affective filter hypothesis captures the relationship between affective variables and the process of L2 acquisition by positing that a variety of affective variables related to success in L2 acquisition (Krashen, 1981). Three major categories emerge: motivation, self-confidence and anxiety. High motivation, a good self-image and low anxiety all contribute positively to reducing or lowering the affective filter through which input must pass on its way to the brain. In this view, input is the primary causative variable in L2 acquisition; affective variables either impede or facilitate the delivery of input to the brain where language-processing occurs.

Relationships between First and Second Language Acquisition Processes

The process of second-language acquisition is not completely different from the development of the first language, but the two processes are not exactly alike either (Fillmore, 1976). As an issue of considerable interest to both researchers and practitioners, the relationship between the processes involved in the development of the bilingual child's languages has been addressed in a number of studies.

In terms of similarity, McLaughlin (1978, p. 206) maintains that both 'first- and second-language acquisition involve essentially the same general (perhaps universal) cognitive strategies'. Research indicates a unity of process that characterises all language acquisition, L1 or L2, and that reflects the use of similar strategies of acquisition in all aspects of communicative competence. Ervin-Tripp (1981) has provided evidence not only that early sentences in a second language are similar in form and function to those of the first language but also that L2 learners are able to bring their conversational knowledge from L1 to bear on acquisition of the new language. This prior knowledge can give older children a significant advantage over L1 learners. With striking frequency, L2 data illustrate parallels with child L1 acquisition. Many of the developmental sequences in syntax, for example, observed for children monolingual in the target language, have also been observed for children acquiring that language as their L2. Simplified word-order structures seen in L1 development are regularly found in L2 data even though the child has acquired more complex structures in L1. Overgeneralisation processes characteristic of L1 acquisition are seen in L2 overgeneralisations of lexical and morphological forms.

Among studies illustrating support for similarities in developmental grammatical sequences between L1 and L2 acquisition is that of Ravem (1975), studying the development of English by his Norwegian-speaking children, ages 3 and 6. In the acquisition of negatives, he found expressions such as 'He not like the house' and 'He don't like it' rather than the forms predicted from Norwegian, 'He like not the house' or 'He like it not.' Studying Spanish-speaking children acquiring English at school, Adams (1978) found that the acquisition of questions and negatives resembled very closely that for English L1 acquisition. *Wh*-questions, for example, fell into three stages of development, from 'What you want?' to overgeneralisation of *be* inversion in 'I don't know where is mines' to, finally, correct use of *be*. *Do*-support emerged in yes/no questions before it appeared in *wh*-questions. Tense was often double-marked as in 'Where did he found it?' All of these structures are typically found in L1 English data.

While research does not support the hypothesis that the acquisition of a second language is identical to that of the first language, neither does it support the position that the two processes are different, as the interference hypothesis based on contrastive analysis of the two languages maintained. As Wode (1981) points out, observed differences in developmental sequences may be due to differences in the total setting in which language acquisition occurs, including cognitive maturity and situational variables. Parallelism between L1 and L2 development may lie in the fact that both employ the same strategies and processes. Basically, it remains to be shown that L2 acquisition is different from L1 acquisition in any fundamental way. Furthermore, the more balanced the input, the more the bilingual child's language acquisition tends to correspond to patterns in monolingual language development (McLaughlin, 1981).

Along with the striking parallels between L1 and L2 acquisition, however, differences can be observed. Second-language learners bring to the task increased experience, including L1 communicative competence, greater levels of cognitive development and maturity. On the one hand, as Fillmore (1976) observes, added age and experience may facilitate the process and, on the other hand, in some ways knowledge of a first language may inhibit it. As she points out, prior knowledge of a first language may lead the child to look for familiar ways of expressing the new language meanings he or she may be accustomed to expressing in L1. This may lead to making distinctions in the L2 that were relevant in the first language but inappropriate in the second. Furthermore, the learner also brings certain attitudes towards the L2 language and culture, ones not yet formed in the young child acquiring L1. Individual characteristics and learning styles which have developed for the older child may serve to inhibit or promote L2 acquisition processes. Personality variables appear to hold special significance for L2 acquisition. For young children this seems to play a less prominent role.

In summary, children acquiring a second langage bring to the task higher degrees of cognitive development, increased age and experience, attitudes towards both their first and second language and culture, their unique set of personality characteristics together with universals functioning in bilingualism (Kessler, 1976). Of the research investigating similarities and differences between L1 and L2 acquisition, most has focused on aspects of grammatical competence, phonology and syntax in particular. Little is yet known about other aspects of communicative competence, similarities and differences in sociolinguistic, discourse and strategic competence. It may be speculated, however, that as more is learned about these components in which many of the aspects are culture-bound, interactions between the processes of transfer from L1 and overgeneralisations in L2 may play a central role.

Simultaneous Bilingualism in Very Young Children

Although much is yet to be learned about how very young children acquire communicative competence in two languages concurrently, carefully detailed diary studies have given insights into the process. One of the classic studies, Leopold's work published in four volumes between 1939 and 1949, documents the development of English and German for his own daughter Hildegard. From his observations certain generalisations emerge and have found support and extensions in subsequent studies.

Input Characteristics and Effects

In the natural environment of becoming bilingual in infancy, two basic patterns of input can be distinguished. In one, the child is presented each language in a one-person, one-language association. In the case of Leopold's Hildegard, English input came from the mother and German input from the father. The second basic pattern is one in which each language is not person specific as happens if one or more caretakers are bilingual and use both languages with the child. The picture becomes further complicated on closer examination. Two types of input may occur. Caretakers may alternate two languages, depending on the nature of the discourse situation, or they may use code-switching within the same discourse. From the same caretaker, consequently, the child may get qualitatively different input of two languages, single-language input determined by discourse occasions and code-switching input on other occasions. Extensive code-switching occurs, for example, among Spanish-English adult bilinguals in the southwestern United States. For many young children this serves as the primary type of input rather than one which clearly distinguishes two language systems.

Another aspect of language input concerns the quantity of input for each language. The language environment may be one which provides a reasonably balanced exposure to the two languages or one which provides higher frequency or greater quantity for one of the languages.

All of these factors interact in complex ways not yet well understood but which can be expected to affect the degree of bilingualism, the rate of realisation of two distinct systems, and the extent of what is sometimes referred to as interference or negative language transfer between the two languages.

However intricate the interaction of input factors in facilitating or inhibiting the development of the two languages, all studies of infant bilingualism give evidence of uneven development of the two languages. One rather obvious generalisation is that children develop faster in the language which is used most in their environment. A completely balanced exposure to two languages is often, if not always, very difficult to maintain in developmental bilingualism. Various researchers have argued that once one language becomes dominant and the other reduced to a subordinate state, interference between the two languages becomes evident (Leopold, 1949a and b; Burling, 1959, for example).

This is a phenomenon more accurately defined as language-mixing (Lindholm and Padilla, 1978). It may happen when one language is spoken in the home and the other is acquired through interaction with playmates (Oksaar, 1976). The greatest amount of mixing seems to occur when the adult input in the child's language environment utilises extensive code-switching. In general, optimal input for reducing mixing appears to be dual language input in the home that consistently associates one person with one language (McLaughlin, 1978). In documenting the bilingual development of his son in Spanish and English, Fantini (1976) gives evidence that the more separate the environments in which each language is used and the more consistent the language use within each of these environments, the more rapidly and more easily bilingual children learn to differentiate their linguistic systems. Close inspection of the nature of mixing indicates that it occurs predominantly at the lexical level (Fantini, 1976; Swain and Wesche, 1975; Cornejo, 1973). An investigation of bilingual mother-child interaction by Garcia and Aguilera (1979) shows that mothers seem to use language-switching as a clarification device and that children tend to mix languages at the lexical level but keep them separate in other components. Much remains to be investigated on the issue of language-mixing in developmental bilingualism.

Language Attitudes

Language input factors, with all of their complexity, further interact with affective or attitudinal factors that the developing bilingual child brings to the language acquisition situation.

The acquisition of two languages depends not only on qualitatively and quantitatively rich language input but also on the child's social needs. These needs frequently lead to attitudes marking each language as necessary or not necessary. Playing with other children assigns the feature of necessary to the language of that social interaction and, commonly for bilingual children, a negative marking is assigned for the language of parents when it differs from that of playmates. Where the social need of a language is minimal, use of that language is reduced. As a result of interaction between balance in language input, social needs for each language, and attitudes that result, among other variables, bilingual children typically go through rejection stages for one of their developing languages. This situation may persist until change occurs in one or more of the variables. Itoh and Hatch (1978) document the rejection stage of Takahiro, age 2;6, whose home language was Japanese. English was reserved to the nursery school where he was enrolled. During his first three months there he played in isolation and would not respond to his English-speaking teacher. English, at least during that period, was not necessary for Takahiro in spite of the surrounding environment. He rejected the English input, making no effort to utilise it socially. Gradually, however, conditions changed. He began to utilise a strategy of repetition, first with adults then with children, mimicking both their language and their behaviour. This active interest in the English around him led to cooperative play and to extensive English-language development. Both the quantity and the quality of English input had shifted dramatically in favour of the acquisition of English.

From studies of developmental bilingualism, a picture emerges that consistently identifies at least two stages by which children become bilingual: the first, an undifferentiated or single-language system; the second, differentiation into two distinct systems.

Stage One: A Single System

Infants who experience dual language input from the onset of language development or before the first-language system is in place appear to form one single language system comprised of elements of both languages. A Spanish-English bilingual child who calls for her *kitty-gato* rather than *kitty-cat* illustrates a combined system in which English *kitty* and Spanish *gato* belong to a single, undifferentiated system. This illustration on the word-forming level is also evident in other components of grammatical competence. At this stage, input is taken from both languages and acted on by cognitive processes to form a single language system. Since it is constructed from elements of two languages, it may be referred to as a mixed language system. Typically, children juxtapose words from both languages in a single utterance as in the mixed Spanish-English utterance 'Have soda en case, Mum?' for 'Can I have soda when we get home, Mum?' or 'Have agua, please?' for 'Can I have some water, please?' Such expressions also illustrate normal developmental syntactic processes for monolinguals, omissions of obligatory function words and morphological markers. On the lexical level, generally children at this stage do not know the names in both languages for an object (Volterra and Taeschner, 1978). Morphologically, they may combine stems from one language with affixes from another (Oksaar, 1976; Burling, 1959).

The pattern for the phonological system at this stage varies with balance between the two languages and normal developmental processes. A number of studies have noted the initial undifferentiated system. Easier sounds to produce will be expected to appear first. Some children seem not to mix sound systems (Oksaar, 1976). In other cases, when one language is dominant, sound features of that language may be substituted for those of the subordinate language (Burling, 1959). At other times, words that contain sounds difficult to produce may systematically be avoided (Celce-Murcia, 1978).

Of significance is the evidence that the undifferentiated system that developing bilingual children construct at this stage is a unique system, distinct from either of the two languages presented to the child. In this way, the process of constructing the undifferentiated or mixed language system parallels the creative construction process that distinguishes the child-language system of the monolingual child from the adult system (Brown, 1973). The development of a bilingual system taps the same basic developmental processes utilised in monolingual development, moving from holophrastic to syntactic, rule-governed utterances. As Titone (1983, p. 175) summarises, 'Generally speaking, it can be said that bilingual development in young children follows an evidently regular course, which is constant throughout different children and different ages.' Both Swain (1972) in her study of French-English bilingual children and Kessler (1971) studying Italian-English bilingual children maintain that the two languages of bilingual children are not encoded separately but rather as a common core of rules. Language-specific rules appear later during the process of language differentiation.

Stage Two: Differentiated Systems

As bilingual children develop, they gradually begin to differentiate between the two language systems. The precise age at which this may occur varies as input conditions, language balance and other linguistic and sociolinguistic variables interact. Fantini (1976), for example, reports the use of distinct, separate language systems by age 2;8 for his son. Imedadze (1967) reports 2;4 Volterra and Taeschner (1978) found age 2;6. At whatever age it occurs, differentiation may be identified when the child starts to use the two languages distinctly to communicate with different people in different languages.

Once the child becomes aware of and differentiates the two language systems, language alternation or code-switching becomes routine, depending on the conditions represented by the person addressed or the specific situations. Bilingual children learn to identify a specific language with a specific person or even age group and with specific situations. Ease of switching depends in large measure on the degree of balance of the two languages. The more that the two languages are equally developed and regularly used, the easier it is to draw on either one. If one is subordinate to the other, the bilingual child exhibits difficulty utilising that language and may experience a peiod of silence until some degree of balance is achieved. In general, however, children whose language is more developed produce fewer mixed utterances than children at earlier stages of development (Redlinger and Park, 1980).

Communicative Competence

Although a complete mapping is not available for each component of communicative competence for children concurrently developing two languages, certain features have been identified.

Grammatical Competence. In separating the two language systems, the developing bilingual must distinguish certain sounds, syntactic structures and lexical items as language-specific. Evidence suggests that development of the phonological system is not significantly different from that for the monolingual child. In addition to mastery of the sound segmentals, the child must also recognise and distinguish the suprasegmental phonemes of each language, the relevant stress, pitch and juncture features. The order of acquisition or differentiation appears to parallel that of L1 monolingual development.

Syntactically, the sequence of development for various grammatical structures appears to follow normal patterns for monolingual children (Carrow, 1971). Kessler (1971) found that simultaneous Italian-English bilingual children acquired structures shared by both languages at approximately the same rate and in the same sequence. A language-specific structure follows later if it is syntactically more complex than a related one in the other language. These findings are consistent with other studies which support the position that bilingual children follow the same basic sequence as monolinguals (Swain, 1972; Mikeš, 1967). Delay in the acquisition of inflectional morphology has been observed in children becoming bilingual, with morphology generally following the development of syntax (Vihman, 1982a; Fantini, 1976; Murrell, 1966). Others have shown no morphological delay (Imedadze, 1967; Burling, 1959). The structure of the languages involved and individual learning strategies may intersect to form differing patterns.

Semantic development parallels that of monolingual development with overextensions frequently occurring, a characteristic of child language. One difficulty for bilinguals is that the meanings of some words have different semantic ranges in the two languages being acquired. For example, *leg* in English applies to both human and animal legs and is distinguished from *foot*. Spanish, however, distinguishes a human leg *pierna* and foot *pie* from an animal leg or foot, *pata*. As the de Villiers (1979, p. 24) point out, 'Children exposed to two or more languages from the beginning tend to be a little slower in their early vocabulary development because each object and event is paired with more than one word. However, they soon catch up with children learning a single language.'

Sociolinguistic Competence. One of the crucial features of simultaneous bilingualism is the acquisition of the rules which distinguish the two languages, permitting the recognition of the appropriateness of one language with a specific person or situation. This competence develops in the stage when the two languages become differentiated.

Discourse Competence. Although much has yet to be mapped out for the simultaneous acquisition of rules governing specific language functions in two languages, one may predict that these rules, like those in other components of competence, parallel those for monolinguals. Research is currently being done in this area.

Strategic Competence. Although relatively little research in simultaneous bilingualism has focused on the cognitive and social strategies outlined by Fillmore (1979) for child L2 learners, anecdotal evidence reveals that children concurrently acquiring two languages employ similar strategies. Following Ventriglia's (1982) taxonomy for strategies which facilitate second-language development, chunking, copy-catting and wearing two hats can be observed in very young bilingual children's efforts to use language in a social situation.

Chunking, a cognitive-developmental strategy, is a strategy by which children imitate phrases or whole utterances which have meaning for them but which are unanalysed and memorised as wholes rather than constructed from constituent parts. It is a strategy which gradually develops (Vihman, 1982b). By using a chunk of meaningful language, children can accomplish communicative goals before they have an internal grammar enabling them to create certain utterances. For example, Itoh and Hatch (1978) document a number of these for Takahiro growing up in Japanese and English environments. Among formulaic chunks actively used were the 'I wanna . . .' and 'I get . . .' patterns. Lita, a Spanish-English bilingual child in Texas observed by Lopez-Schule (1982) made extensive use of the same 'I wanna . . .' pattern in both English and Spanish, 'Yo quiero . . .', at the early stage of differentiating her two languages around age 2;9.

Copy-catting, a social-affective strategy, allows children to imitate in role-play another person by copying both their verbal and non-verbal behaviour. Takahiro's efforts to imitate other children in the nursery school, a strategy which had facilitative effects on the acquisition of English, is an example of this strategy.

The bilingual-bicultural strategy of wearing two hats employs a strategy of code-switching, usually done spontaneously, to convey cultural or social meaning. It can be a conscious or unconscious selection of language variants, taking into account the social situation and the child's relation to the listener. Lita, at age 2;3, gives an example of this strategy in the following conversation with her mother:

Mother: ¿Qué quieres, Lita? Quieres leche?
(What do you want, Lita? Do you want some milk?)
Child: No leche.
Mother: ¿Quieres agua? (Do you want some water?)
Child: No agua.
Mother: ¿Quieres jugo? (Do you want some juice?)
Child: No jugo, Candy, mamí.
Mother: No candy, no, Lita.
Child: Candy! (with great emphasis, followed by a long pause)
. . . Dame dulce, please. (Give me candy, please.)

The language switch from English to Spanish in asking for candy took place in a very slow, deliberate manner, evidently with the expectation that the situation to bring about the realisation of candy called for Spanish.

Strategic competence plays a central role in drawing children into the social situations which ultimately provide the input necessary to trigger language acquisition processes.

Awareness of Two Languages

The point at which bilingual children acquiring two languages simultaneously develop a metalinguistic awareness of their two languages varies individually but appears to develop before the school years. In another conversation with her mother, Lita at age 3;6 gave the first indication that she had an awareness of her access to two languages. After asking Lita to give several examples of Spanish and English words, the following exchange occurs:

Mother: ¿ Tu sabes hablar mucho o poquito inglés?
(Can you speak a lot or a little bit of English?)
Child: Mucho inglés.
Mother: ¿ Y tu sabes hablar mucho o poquito español?
(And can you speak a lot or a little bit of Spanish?)
Child: Mucho español.
Mother: ¿ Y oyes, Lita, a ti te gusta hablar el inglés o el español o los dos? (And tell me, Lita, do you like to speak English or Spanish or both?)
Child: Dos. (holds up two fingers)
That's inglés. (points to one finger)
And that's español! (points to another finger)

Of critical importance is an understanding of the fragility of bilingualism for very young children. Removed from a bilingual input and the need to draw on the two language systems for social interactions, a bilingual child can soon lose one of the languages (Elliot, 1981). Burling's Garo-English bilingual son lost Garo within six months of leaving India even though he had used it for two years, from ages 1;4 to 3;4. On the other hand, continued input can stabilise the bilingualism, allowing for distinct separate language use as it did for Leopold's Hildegard by age 7, when she could keep her German and English bilingualism separated even though her English was dominant over her German. To be maintained, bilingualism requires the continued use of both languages in communicative naturalistic settings.

Sequential Bilingualism in Preschool Children

At about three years of age children normally have developed basic communicative competence in their first language. Refinements in the various components – grammatical, sociolinguistic, discourse, strategic – continue to take place during the school years. However, in the preschool period children have extensive access to language. To undertake the process of acquiring another language around age 3 is to add a second language to that already basically in place, to engage in the process occurring in informal environments when attention is directed to the meaning of utterances rather than to their linguistic form. It is this process which preschool children utilise exclusively in developing a second language (Krashen, 1982). As such, it draws on the causative variables of language input provided by the environment and the affective filter variables the child brings to the situation. Contrary to popular views, not all children acquire a second language successfully or with ease. When input is deficient, in quality or in quantity, or when children, because of the complex set of personality characteristics each brings to the task, have negative attitudes or do not have access to the cognitive and social strategies that facilitate language acquisition, the process may be greatly impaired. If children are put on the defensive by being required to perform too early in the L2, the process can be interrupted or slowed down. Other children actively processing the new language input may utilise a long 'silent period' during which they do not verbally perform in the second language, a situation which may give a misreading on the nature of their bilingualism.

Although recent research has increasingly focused on the process of language acquisition and the variables the learner brings to the process, it nevertheless can be useful to examine aspects of the system the learner constructs for gaining further insights into the process.

The product of the L2 acquisition process is generally referred to as an interlanguage (Selinker, 1972; Corder, 1981). It is a unique system constructed by the child from the portion of L2 input that the brain acts on, the intake. The interlanguage is a dynamic, fluid system, shifting and changing as the child reorganises it to accommodate new rules. A developmental continuum, the interlanguage is characterised by the so-called errors which mark divergence from the native-speaker norms for the target language. Traditionally, this continuum is segmented into broad stages – beginning, intermediate, advanced – which roughly take into account how closely the interlanguage approximates the native-speaker system. In this view, the making of errors plays an inevitable and necessary role for the successful outcome of the L2 process. Errors are a function of the process. Rather than serving as indicators of failure, they provide evidence of the learner's acquisition strategies.

Developmental Stages

Unlike simultaneous bilingualism, which takes as its starting point the onset of language or an early point in child language, sequential bilingualism takes as its starting point the L1 system. Recent research indicates that this system is drawn upon primarily in the early stages of L2 development. As the process continues, the L1 has less influence and the errors observed in the interlanguage resemble increasingly the normal, developmental errors characterising children's acquisition of the target language as their L1. Aspects of interaction between the child's L1 and L2 may continue, however, throughout the development of the second language. Interference, utilisation of rules from L1 in the developing L2 system, does occur but less extensively than assumed in the past. In other words, children appear to follow their own built-in syllabus which resembles in large measure, although not identically, that of children acquiring the target language as their L1. As a result, errors tend to be similar for all children acquiring the same L2 even though their first languages differ. Some evidence for this is seen in a series of morpheme studies conducted with children from diverse first languages acquiring English as their second language (Burt and Dulay, 1980). Furthermore, errors that children make appear to be remarkably similar to those made by adults learning the same L2.

Developmental stages may be defined in terms of the rules acquired in the L2. Meisel and his colleagues (1981) argue, however, that L2 acquisition is not a linear process, following a straight line from the starting point to proficiency in the target language. Although they do not exclude the possibility that there are developmental stages identified in terms of rules emerging in a predictable order, they point out that the notion of developmental stage must allow the possibility of considerable variation within a stage and the notion that changes in the developing system do not necessarily indicate a new stage of development. Moreover, there is no reason to assume that the process of L2 acquisition in a natural setting necessarily starts with 'easy' rules, holding the 'hard' rules for a later stage. Rules develop as a result of communicative needs, not linguistic difficulty. As a result, a complex rule with high probability of error may be acquired early but used deviantly over a long period of time. Other rules, of course, might be applied correctly from the beginning.

Longitudinal studies with corroborative cross-sectional studies of L2 learners provide insights into developmental stages. However, the process of L2 acquisition is not simply that of acquiring an increasing number of rules. Over time, in the process of adding new rules, some are dropped and others changed. Analysis of the grammatical complexity of a language sample from any one learner does not give sufficient information to determine the specific developmental stage at that time. Furthermore, language does not develop uniformly in all components. Progress in one area does not imply similar developments in all others. Assessment of developmental stages is further complicated by the fact that, in the effort to communicate, a second language learner does not necessarily reveal the highest level of development of the system. The need to get a message across may lead to certain strategic shortcuts that obscure the system's highest level of development.

Communicative Competence

Much is yet to be investigated on children's development of L2 communicative competence. Nevetheless, certain observations can give insights into processes for sequential bilingualism.

Grammatical Competence. In acquiring rules of phonology, morphology, syntax and semantics, children developing a second language engage in a type of 'juggling act', acquiring portions of each component in a kind of multidimensional fashion with elements of each component undergoing acquisition simultaneously.

The amount of influence that the L1 exerts on L2 acquisition has received considerable research attention in which two competing hypotheses are readily discernible. The developmental hypothesis takes the position that L2 acquisition closely parallels L1 development. Language transfer from L1 to L2 assumes only a minor role. Conversely, the transfer hypothesis holds that the L1 system affects the acquisition of the L2. In its strong version, difficulties can be predicted by a contrastive analysis of the two language systems. These difficulties result from negative transfer or interference from the L1. Little empirical evidence supports this strong position but research does support a role for transfer in the second-language acquisition process.

Evaluating the development of phonology for an Icelandic child, age 6, acquiring English as a second language in a naturalistic setting, Hecht and Mulford (1982) found that neither the developmental hypothesis nor the transfer hypothesis alone explained the course of English phonological development. Rather, a systematic interaction between both positions accounted best for the acquisition order observed. They hypothesised a continuum for the role of transfer and normal L1 developmental processes for the target language in the following continuum:

transfer dominant ⟷ developmental processes dominant

vowels — liquids — stops — fricatives and affricates

Variability in the sources of language input is a complicating factor in analysis of phonological development. Additionally, children often show an early awareness of the new phonological system, frequently playing at 'speaking' the second language when, in fact, they are using their L1 but adopting features of the L2. Acquisition of the phonological system in child second-language acquisition is a far more complex process than often assumed. 'Learning to speak without an accent may look like child's play, but, in fact, it is a complex process which we are just beginning to understand' (Hecht and Mulford, 1982, p. 327).

Much of the study of child L2 acquisition has focused on morphology and syntax. Studies on the L2 acquisition order of selected English morphemes presents consistent regularities for speakers of different first languages but does not parallel exactly the developmental order for the L2. Dulay and Burt (1974) found differences from L1 English orders for Spanish- and Cantonese-speaking children, Fathman (1975) for Korean- and Spanish-speaking groups, and Kessler and Idar (1977, 1979) for a Vietnamese-speaking child. The developmental sequence observed for these children does not overrule the fact that individual children take different routes in acquiring the system, displaying the within-stage variation expected for the L2 process. In the area of syntax, a major area of L2 research with children has focused on the development of the auxiliary system, which includes negation, yes/no questions, *wh*-questions, and *do*-support in negatives and questions. Another area investigated includes acquisition of relative clauses and tests of the minimal distance principle, which examines noun-verb connections and pronoun reference. For a fuller picture of the second-language sequencing of syntactic structures, studies are needed which address a much broader range of structures. Of importance, too, is the observation by Wagner-Gough (1978) that the emergence of a linguistic form may occur prior to its function, an issue little investigated. In studying data from Homer, a 5-year-old, Wagner-Gough noted that the pattern for acquisition of the progressive *-ing* followed closely that for L1 English but he had no awareness of the tense/aspect function of *going, go, I'm go, I going* and *I go*, used in semantic free variation to signal movement from one place to another in the present, past, future. Such form-function relationships form essential units for development of the semantic system as well as the syntax.

Just as studies of L1 acquisition of vocabulary show extensive individual variation so, too, do those which have examined L2 development. Yoshida (1978) found that the Japanese-English bilingual child he studied, age 3;5, acquired more nominals than other classes during a seven-month period. Items from semantic categories that closely related to the child's world were acquired first: lexical items for food, animals, vehicles, outdoor objects. English vocabulary was also expanded through loanwords taken into Japanese from English. As children's life experiences vary, the range of vocabulary may also be expected to vary.

Sociolinguistic Competence. Rules for using language appropriately begin development at a very early age in young children's L1. Bates (1976) has shown that even before age 2 children can express a particular function of language with a variety of forms. Around age 2;6 they learn to soften imperative force with *please*, for example. By about age 3 they know how to increase the degree of politeness even further. However, since development of this type of pragmatic competence also closely parallels cognitive development, many of the refinements in rules governing appropriate social use of language do not occur until the school years.

Preschool children engaging in L2 acquisition processes can be expected to bring sociolinguistic sensitivity to the new language. However, acquisition of the necessary forms to carry out specific functions in a variety of ways and an awareness of the social significance of specific forms is a complex process that, as for monolingual children, requires further cognitive growth occurring during the school years along with increased proficiency in the new language system. From a second-language perspective, certain aspects of linguistic and functional rules governing appropriate language use may be culture-specific as well as language-specific. It may be in this area, in particular, that L1 interference plays its most active role. Second-language learners may expect to find equivalent expressions in the new language governed by the familiar L1 set of social norms. Nevertheless, as Blum-Kukla (1982, p. 53) observes, 'the complex nature of the interdependence between pragmatic linguistic and social factors in the target language will often prevent him from getting his meaning across'.

Discourse Competence. From the earliest beginnings of L2 development, children are engaged in the structuring of discourse. Their conversational partners may be caretakers or other children. In either case, topics must be nominated and understood, turns taken, information given, clarifications sought, comments made. Saying something relevant is one of the first rules of conversation. Data from children acquiring a second language show these efforts from the beginning, even when they do not have the necessary vocabulary or structures to do it clearly. Strategies relying on non-verbal means or simple repetitions of something said by the conversational partner may be the only means available to accomplish this but it is in the effort to carry on the conversation that syntax is built up and progress made in L2 development, not the reverse (Hatch, 1983).

In child-child discourse, one dimension of being relevant not present in child-adult interactions is language play, a non-literal, rule-bound use of language. In Peck's (1980) analysis, children acquiring a second language not only engage in the process but appear to develop language from it. She suggests that the kinds of practice opportunities for the sounds and forms of the L2 and the intense affective climate that accompanies this type of conversation contribute productively to L2 development. Children attend to each other's utterances intensely and put pressure on each other to continue contributing to the language play activity. Another dimension of child-child discourse is that of the language of games in which chunks quickly learned and used repetitively appear as in *my turn*, *give it to me*, *throw it to me*, *I won*. Access to these chunks contributes to involvement in the social interaction with other children. This facilitates the input necessary for further L2 acquisition.

Strategic Competence. When children are confronted with unfamiliar input, they draw on one of the fundamental properties of learning, formation of expectancies based on prior experience. Keller-Cohen (1981) presents evidence that one of the strategies children acquiring a second language employ, in addition to using their general knowledge of the world and contextual cues, is to search for structural similarities between the familiar L1 and the unfamiliar L2. This might also be described as an aspect of what Ventriglia (1982) calls bridging, a cognitive-developmental strategy through which children appear to tie words to concepts they already know in their L1, one of the first clearly observable strategies children employ in L2 acquisition.

From the bridging strategy, children move to chunking, use of formulaic expressions as unanalysed wholes. The most detailed study of this strategy is in Fillmore's (1976) study of five Spanish-speaking children, ages 7,7, acquiring English. Observing the individual variation apparent in this group, she emphasises the vital function formulas serve in opening communication channels with L2 speakers, gaining access to crucial L2 input with expressions as *lookit*, *you know what?*, *I wanna play*. The most effective L2 learner in the group, Nora, not only used chunks extensively but also learned rapidly to analyse them to get frames she could use productively, the strategy of creating. These strategies served Nora well in becoming a part of the social group that spoke her new language. Fillmore concludes that the strategy of acquiring chunks or formulaic speech is central to L2 acquisition.

Following Ventriglia (1982), social-affective strategies children use in meaningful interactions in their new language are listening to others and sometimes trying to repeat, guessing and making inferences, code-switching, role-playing. Learning style strategies include beading, a style based on a need to learn one word at a time because of the importance attached to meaning; braiding, a style in which the learner attends to the context of chunks and the relationships among them; orchestrating, a style in which the learner places much emphasis on sounds and repetition of sounds. Children may combine all three learning style strategies in the L2 process. Motivational style strategies play a role in prompting the use of certain social-affective strategies. In the first, crystallising, children initially reject the second language and culture, maintaining their own. In cross-over, the preference is for the L2 language and culture over the first. Through the third motivational style, criss-crossing, children choose to identify with both languages and cultures.

Through the various strategies available, children can successfully enter into conversations, the basic building blocks of language development.

Sequential Bilingualism in School-age Children

Although much of the process of L2 acquisition remains the same for preschool and school-age children, certain differences also need to be taken into account. Increased age, cognitive maturity and more extensive language experience are variables which can serve to enhance the process. Other variables which play a critical role are differences in the language environment, including the kinds of language input and the structuring of the classroom setting, together with the affective environment created and the more highly developed affective filters children bring to the situation. At school, too, a heightened metalinguistic awareness of language is developed as children are taught to become aware of language as a separate entity. Perhaps most crucially, however, a major difference is in the definition of second-language proficiency. This involves essentially orality, listening and speaking, for preschoolers but, additionally, literacy, reading and writing, for school-age L2 learners.

Language Environment

Language at school in many ways differs from language outside the classroom, at home and at play. Not only does it include much new content but also it is used to develop new competencies in an array of cognitive processes. The highly context-bound oral out-of-school language gives way to what, with increasing frequency, is highly decontextualised language as children learn to read and rely on reading for much of their learning. New types of discourse appear in the teaching-learning process. New styles of using language, even the spoken language, may be required. These and other factors combine to provide differences in the language input from what younger children generally experience in preschool years. For school-age children beginning L2 acquisition, these differences compound the task of developing a new language. Informal, out-of-class varieties of the L2 are needed to interact socially with peers. At the same time, a more formal, language-at-school variety is needed for school success. For the total range of a second language to develop, a rich, varied input is needed to facilitate development in all aspects of the L2 needed for success, socially and academically. The quantity and quality of the input available and the extent to which each child can make use of it are affected by a multiplicity of factors. The school's way of structuring the input and the child's own set of characteristics brought to the L2 task interact in complex ways to facilitate or inhibit the process.

Although affective variables play a role in even young children's bilingual development, they may exert stronger effects with increasing age and maturity. Attitudes towards the new language and culture are crucial variables. In addition, they may interact with the affective climate set in the classroom by the teacher. Negative responses in any of these dimensions can inhibit the L2 process just as very positive ones can promote it (Fillmore, 1979).

Relationships between the classroom structure, including the instructional style of open classrooms with many learning centres as opposed to more traditional teacher-centred arrangements, and the composition of the class in terms of the ratio of L2 learners to native speakers, are crucial variables which interact with the individual variation among L2 learners, as Fillmore's (1983) longitudinal research project with young school children shows. A relatively open class structure works only if there are enough native speakers of the target language in the class to allow for the necessary sustained interactions with the L2 learners to make enough input possible. In such a classroom setting, however, the amount of language as input to any individual child will depend on the child's own ability to seek out the children in the class who speak the target language and to get into some kind of sustained interaction with them. Because of each child's unique set of personality characteristics, not all children can do this. For classrooms in which the concentration of L2 learners is high, a more teacher-centred structuring is necessary to ensure adequate input. Success depends in large measure on the teacher's own sensitivity to each child's level of proficiency and to knowing how to make the modifications necessary to ensure comprehensible input for each child. Even though the orientation may be teacher-directed, the teacher, nevertheless, must manage to interact with the children individually with enough frequency to make L2 development possible. Again, the classroom setting interacts with the individual's characteristics. As a result, some children are successful L2 learners; others are not.

Individual differences themselves result from interactions between the nature of the task of acquiring a second language, the strategies needed for the task, and the personal characteristics of the learner (Fillmore, 1979). When these differences interact with variations in the classroom setting, the development of a second language at school becomes a highly intricate process.

In an experimental programme using peer tutoring, Johnson (1983) found positive effects on social interaction and English as a second-language proficiency for a group of Spanish-speaking children paired with fluent English-speakers. The increased verbal interaction and vocabulary comprehension in English pointed out the importance of utilising the language input of fluent target-language speakers in designing L2 programmes. Also important in the school setting is allowance for a 'silent period' during which the L2 is developing but the length of which may vary markedly among children (Day, 1981).

As part of the schooling process, children grow in a metalinguistic awareness of language. This perhaps marks the most general difference between child L1 and L2 development (McLaughlin, 1982). Children acquiring the L2 in school already know, at least in a general way, what language is. However, as they develop cognitively, they also can benefit from overt, explicit focus on language form. This is the process of language-learning, distinguished from the natural process of language acquisition (Krashen, 1981). It is not available to young children since it rests on various analytical abilities that come with cognitive growth during the school years.

Second-language Proficiency in School Contexts

The communicative competence framework is useful in describing the acquisition of a second language provided that it takes into account developmental perspectives applicable to children, recognising that certain aspects of each component are mastered early and others not until well into the school years, even for native speakers. In addition, it is necessary to consider what constitutes L2 proficiency in school contexts and how the L1 and L2 are developmentally related, particularly as this affects language at school.

To distinguish linguistic demands at school from those of interpersonal contexts outside of school, Cummins (1980a, 1981) conceptualises communicative proficiency along two continuums. One continuum relates to the range of contextual support available to the language users. On the one end, context-embedded communication relies strongly on paralinguistic and situational cues to language use, basic interpersonal communication skills (BICS) involving face-to-face language encounters. On the other end of the continuum, language is primarily context-reduced, relying essentially on linguistic cues to meaning involved in cognitive/academic language proficiency (CALP), the literacy-related aspects of language use. The second continuum addresses the developmental aspects of communicative competence in terms of the degree of cognitive demands imposed by the task or activity. Initial L1 acquisition, for example, is cognitively demanding and, at the same time, context-embedded. Preschoolers eventually are able to use cognitive-embedded language in a cognitively undemanding way. Second-language acquisition, in initial stages at least, is cognitively demanding, involving for school-age children both context-embedded and context-reduced language use. These varieties correspond to interpersonal oral language on the one hand and literacy-related language on the other. Academic success at school requires utilisation of context-reduced, cognitively demanding literacy-related tasks in which L2 users must be able to participate actively.

Cummins argues that CALP is cross-lingual, that once acquired elements are applicable in any language context, L1 or L2. In other words, once this aspect of language proficiency is mastered in L1, it will manifest itself in L2 once enough of the L2 code is available. This explains why older second-language learners whose L1 CALP is more highly developed may manifest CALP more rapidly in their second language than younger children whose L1 CALP is less developed. For children who come to the L2 acquisition task with CALP already well developed in L1, the L2 realisation is highly favoured. For those, however, who have little or no L1 CALP, the process is further complicated, as the language interdependence hypothesis formulated by Cummins (1979) states.

Learning a second language for school use is a task that imposes its own specific demands, teaching the child to become aware of language as a separate structure and to use it in context-reduced forms where the meaning must be taken from the printed page without other cues or written down in such a form that the reader can take the message accurately without recourse to contexts available through face-to-face encounters of spoken language. Differentiation between context-embedded and context-reduced and cognitively demanding and cognitively undemanding tasks outlines a critical distinction between L2 development in the preschool years and L2 development at school.

Summary

Children may develop communicative competence in two languages from the onset of language development, simultaneous bilingualism, or after the first language is in place, sequential bilingualism. In either case, the communicative competence framework for second-language proficiency provides a theoretical basis for studying the processes of language acquisition in bilingual children. Acquisition of communicative competence recognises and distinguishes development in four components: (1) grammatical competence for mastery of the language code; (2) sociolinguistic competence for mastery of appropriate language use in various sociolinguistic contexts; (3) discourse competence for mastery of how to combine meanings and forms to achieve unity in a specific mode of communication such as a conversation; (4) strategic competence for mastery of verbal and non-verbal strategies to compensate for breakdowns in communication or to enhance communicative effectiveness.

This sketch of language acquisition processes in bilingual children outlines similarities and differences in basic processes accounting for monolingual and bilingual language development. It further distinguishes children developing two languages simultaneously from language onset from those developing two languages sequentially. The latter are further differentiated for preschool and school-year contexts for second-language acquisition. Emphasis is given to the role of the language environment, the input available, and the individual variables children bring to the process of acquiring communicative competence in two languages. To understand fully the acquisition of bilingualism in children, the developmental perspectives of communicative competence for very young children, older preschool children, and school-age children together with relationships between bilingual children's two languages and aspects of communicative competence related to school contexts must all be taken into account. Becoming bilingual is a uniquely human phenomenon that is extraordinarily complex.

3 BILINGUALISM AND COGNITIVE DEVELOPMENT

Sandra Ben-Zeev

In trying to understand the relationship between bilingualism and cognition as well as the relationship between language handicap and cognition we must first confront the problem of definition, or at least realise that it exists. There are different kinds of bilingualism, depending on the conditions under which the second language arises and the age at which it arises. The term 'language handicap' has a certain indeterminacy about it, and probably encompasses several different conditions.

Concerning bilingualism, when the second language is initiated by the school, as in a language immersion programme, this creates one kind of bilingualism. When both languages arise at a much younger age, but under conditions in which the interlocutors or contexts or topics are kept clearly separate, this is another kind of bilingualism. This, in turn, is to be distinguished from the situation in which the child experiences language-switching in his environment from a very young age, i.e. a given caretaker switches from one language to the other in talking to the child.

Concerning language handicap, even when we clearly distinguish between a specific language handicap and general mental retardation, by specifying that the IQ of the language-handicapped child should be 'normal', the manner in which we measure intelligence makes a difference. Should we measure just performance IQ? If we go further and specify that verbal IQ should be normal too, then we are likely to define a group whose handicap is relatively mild. If we equate only performance IQ, then what is to distinguish the resultant 'language handicap' group from verbally-retarded individuals? One way out of this is to use a battery of tests, all of which are related to intelligence but which consist of separate tests of quite specific skills. The overall scores can be used to evaluate the extent to which the suspected 'language-retarded' individuals are similar in intelligence to other children. Particular subtests which, after being separately treated as independent variables, prove to be significantly related to the language handicap itself, can be used diagnostically, but not counted as part of the intelligence battery for purposes of equating the language-handicapped individuals with normal individuals on intelligence.

Finding such related 'IQ' subtests would help us determine the nature of the language handicap. Also, treating intelligence in this way will allow a finer distinction within the sphere of 'verbal IQ'.

Most studies which relate bilingualism to language handicaps do not define intelligence this carefully. In fact, most studies which try to determine the consequences of language handicap are only correlational, so even without bilingualism as a complicating factor, it is difficult to determine causation.

The problem, however, is not just one of methodology. For example, an important problem is how to interpret vocabulary deficit. Vocabulary scores have been found to be closely related to Spearman's 'g' or general intelligence factor, and often vocabulary tests such as the Peabody Vocabulary Test are used as measures of general intelligence. Yet, reduced vocabulary has been found to be an accompaniment of reading deficiency, which is the measure of language handicap used in a great many studies (see Vellutino's review, 1980). Reduced vocabulary has also been found to be an accompaniment of bilingualism, whether the bilinguals show quite high levels of language-processing (Ben-Zeev, 1972; Rosenblum and Pinker, 1983) or lower levels (Ben-Zeev, 1975).

There can be many different reasons for vocabulary deficit, and it is likely that the reason in the case of the bilinguals is different from that in the case of the language disabled. The reason in the case of the bilinguals may be simply a matter of reduced experience. The bilinguals hear fewer references to any particular word in their environment because they must share their conversations between two language systems, and thus they are less familiar with any given word. However, it may also be a more direct result of the bilingualism. As will be discussed later in this chapter, Talmy (1984) claims that verbs of a particular language tend to incorporate within them elements which are characteristic of the syntax of that language. This may mean that a verb in language A which has the same rough meaning as its counterpart in language B will be inhibited from connecting associatively with its counterpart in language B because of the incompatible syntactic element it contains. The language A verb is associated with one cognitive-syntactic strategy, whereas the language B verb is associated with another. Cowan and Sarmed (1976) have shown that in reading a second language, confusions often arise as a result of the reader's making predictions based on cognitive strategies in language A. One way that the bilingual can ward off this kind of deficit is to put up some kind of barrier to interlingual semantic association. This, in turn, would result in narrow semantic categories associated with words and lower vocabulary. Under this scenario, there would be an inverse relationship between vocabulary deficit and reading skill for the bilingual. The devices which serve to defend against interlingual interference in reading – devices which perhaps are used by the better bilinguals, who are more aware of the potential interference and its causes than less skilled bilinguals – may be the cause of low vocabulary. At this point there is no evidence for this hypothesis, but it would explain why even highly skilled bilinguals have shown vocabulary deficit.

As for less skilled bilinguals, there is some evidence that they may manifest lower verbal academic skills generally, so that the vocabulary deficit could be considered merely a part of that general verbal deficit. Many early studies gave this result, but these results must be discounted because of the gross failure of essential controls in these studies. A more recent study by Tsushima and Hogan (1975) found a similar result for Japanese-English bilinguals in grades 4 and 5, as compared to a monolingual control group matched in non-verbal IQ. However, this study could have been still more precise about the nature of the bilingualism of those children, so this result is still uncertain.

In the case of language-handicapped children, the reasons for the vocabulary deficit could also be various. It could be that inefficiency in decoding may, over a long period, result in low vocabulary. Perfetti and Lesgold (1978) posit that the poor reader has difficulty in naming a word stimulus and in retrieving semantic information in response to a name.

The cause of the vocabulary deficit may also, however, be much more deeply concerned with lexical organisation. Miller (1969) views the lexicon as organised not only on the basis of semantic features but also on the basis of information about the grammatical relationships into which given words may enter. Thus, a given lexical item may belong to the noun class, and it may further be classifiable as human, animate, inanimate, etc. It is classifiable by the inclusion relationships it can enter, potential part-whole relationships, and functional relationships. All such information may be coded along with a given word and may determine its position in a hierarchical structure of words in an associational network as well as its potential position within a sentence. The language-disabled child may be deficient in the development of this lexical organisation system.

Given all these different possible reasons for a finding of poor vocabulary, we may conclude that: (1) it is not a simple thing to control for IQ or to 'equate' IQ in testing hypotheses concerning how language deficit and bilingualism interact; and (2) in order to understand any possible interactions we must go much more deeply into testing possible reasons, based upon the kind of explanations noted above.

What is likely to be the explanation for poor vocabulary in the case of a language-disabled bilingual child? The combination of the two conditions reduces the number of reasons we need consider. The situation of lowered vocabulary as a kind of adaptive mechanism to reduce interlingual interference on the part of the bilingual is not likely to occur in the case where the bilingual is language disabled. This is because adaptive measures to prevent interference are likely to occur for a bilingual who has some consciousness of languages as systems. A bilingual who is language disabled is unlikely to have this consciousness. His interpretation of a word in isolation is less likely to contain its relationship to syntactic position. His interpretation of a word within ongoing speech is likely to be dependent upon support from the global situational context but relatively little from the purely linguistic syntax or discourse structure. Therefore, his responses are less likely to be affected by considerations of possible interference from the structure of the other language.

Vellutino (1980, pp. 264-91) concluded from his review of research on dyslexia that there is much to support the notion of language handicap as involving reduced ability to process syntax. There are undoubtedly other factors involved as well, but a considerable number of research studies concur that there is some inefficiency in syntactic processing. One set of studies that seem to contradict this finding (Perfetti and Lesgold, 1978) found that the performance of poor readers was negatively affected by scrambling of sentences which destroys syntactic predictability. This implies that the poor readers had depended upon the syntactic organisation of the intact sentence. But the degree of handicap of these subjects may have been mild, compared to that of the subjects on which the findings were made concerning syntactic processing difficulty.

In trying to determine how possible cognitive deficiencies which accompany language handicap interact with the effects of bilingualism, I will concentrate on two cognitive factors which are important to both. These are: (1) the ability to understand language as a system, in terms of syntactic structure; (2) the ability to take different perspectives. The latter manifests itself within language in the form of understanding of the sequencing of sentences in a discourse so as to accommodate the perspective of the hearer. It is also manifest in the extent to which the speaker adjusts his rhetorical style to fit the particular needs of the speaker and of the situation.

The following section reviews studies of bilingualism as developed in immersion school settings and in more natural settings to investigate the question of how this relates to the understanding of language as a system, and of how this might relate to language retardation. A later section concerns perspective-taking.

Positive, 'Neutral' and Negative Effects of Bilingualism in Immersion School Situations and in Natural Situations

Cummins (1976, 1979) has gathered together research findings from different types of bilingual situations under a threshold theory of bilingualism effects. According to this theory, whether bilingualism has positive, neutral or negative effects on cognition depends on the extent to which the bilingual has achieved understanding of his language as a system. The level of understanding is conceived of as an intervening variable which is affected by a number of different factors including, in addition to intelligence and native ability, various socio-economic and cultural factors which affect the child's understanding of his languages mainly through affecting his attitude towards learning them. As for the level of understanding of language achieved, no particular level is specified, because it depends upon the level required by the environment, but it is understood that schooling, in the later grades especially, requires a 'cognitive-academic' type of language understanding, which operates without strong support from the immediate context and which is relatively self-conscious. Two threshold levels are tentatively posited. The lower threshold level is that level of language functioning which is adequate for the needs of the environment. In the case of children in language immersion programmes, the environment is that of the school and school work. If, for whichever reason, the child has not achieved a level of functioning in his first language adequate for the needs of the school, he will be handicapped in learning the second language, the language of school immersion. The result will be a deficit to the child: his first language will suffer because it does not have the added experience in the school context for it to develop, and the second language cannot develop adequately until a certain level of decontextualisation has been reached with the first. The child's work will suffer because the work is presented in L2, which is not developed sufficiently in the child to be used as an adequate vehicle for learning.

Above that threshold, it is hypothesised, effects on general cognition are neutral. That is, the child will learn L2 sufficiently to carry on school work in that language and to speak it fluently, albeit not as well as a native speaker, and his L1, except for a temporary period during which the school postpones teaching reading in L1 for a few years, will show no deficit. Once reading is finally taught in L1, the child learns it easily, having mastered the basic skill in the course of learning how to read in L2. The effect of the bilingualism on the other subject matter and on the level of language-processing itself is neutral.

Achieving the lower threshold of bilingual competence would be sufficient to avoid any negative cognitive effects, but if the attainment of a second, higher threshold of bilingual competence is achieved, it will lead to accelerated cognitive growth.

Concerning failure to achieve the lower threshold, the situation of working-class children from Finnish immigrant families in Sweden is a clear case. These children, some of whom were born in Sweden, do poorly in school when taught exclusively through the medium of Swedish. On test results they show poor cognitive performance on Swedish language tests, and their Finnish language is below the level of comparable children in Finland. Skutnabb-Kangas and Toukomaa (1976) use the word 'semilingualism' to describe this condition of poor mastery of both languages relative to native speakers of comparable social class, poor understanding of the meanings of abstract concepts, of synonyms, and poor vocabulary in general.

'Semilingualism' does not imply failure to communicate in ordinary everyday concrete situations. In fact, the Finnish children themselves, their parents and their teachers judge them to be quite fluent. The idea is that this fluency is only superficial and masks a deficit in the knowledge of the structure of both languages.

In this case the factors which are presumed to cause this result are attitudinal. The Finnish-origin children are not economically deprived, living as they do in a socialist country, nor do they suffer from deprivation of stimulating play materials or nursery school experience (Skutnabb-Kangas and Toukomaa, 1980). The working-class orientation of the parents is presumed to accompany a relative lack of interest in language as such, and lack of emphasis on verbalisation in child-parent interaction. The group as a whole is emotionally attached to the mother country rather than Sweden or the Swedish language. They travel to nearby Finland several times a year, and the majority hope to return to live in Finland. This pattern is thought to foster poor motivation to learn Swedish in school, with resulting poor performance. According to the authors, when 'language shelter' programmes were instituted to teach Finnish children in the early school years in the Finnish language, their performance greatly improved in both languages, and also their school work.

Cummins believes that a similar explanation holds for why children who enter English-speaking schools in the United States from lower-class Spanish-speaking minority groups have problems. The social class and attitudinal factors impede their learning of English, while the fact that the native language is a minority language with low status in the larger society contributes to its decline in their speech. The result is what Lambert (1975) calls 'subtractive bilingualism', in which the situation retards the development of both languages, or else it results in loss of one of them. 'Additive bilingualism', on the other hand, is a situation in which the bilingual's first language is dominant in the environment, as in the case of immersion programmes in French for English-speakers in Canada, or where the first language is at least prestigious, so there is no danger that learning the second will threaten the strength of the first language. In this case, according to the theory, the bilingual adds another language to his repertory of skills at no cost to his competence in his L1. This situation is said to characterise the school language immersion programmes in Canada, which primarily concern middle-class children who are secure in their dominant English language and whose parents are very approving of the idea of their children learning French in the school immersion programme. This provides incentive to learn the second language with no discouragement of the first. It was found that introduction of L2 as the language of the classroom in kindergarten and continuing all subject matter except formal study of English in this language, including reading, had no detrimental effects on the English L1, nor did it create any deficit in L1 reading or other functioning when L1 reading was finally introduced in later grades. On arithmetic and most other content matter taught in French, these children were found to do as well as their monolingual English-speaking counterparts in those subjects taught in English. As for more general cognitive tests, no differences were found for these children on tests involving convergent thinking or abstraction. Tests of divergent thinking on children in situations such as these show contradictory results; the Canadian immersion students sometimes test higher on such tests, but Torrance *et al.* (1970) found a deficit for children in a similar situation on fluency and flexibility aspects of divergent thinking together with better performance on originality. Other studies which show some kind of positive association between bilingualism and divergent thinking are Bruck, Lambert and Tucker (1976); Carringer (1974); Cummins and Gulutsan (1974); Landry (1974); and Scott (1973). Details of the language-learning situation were not given in the Torrance study, and the causes of the difference are not clear. Cummins concludes that, on the whole, the results for more general cognitive functioning as the result of the immersion experience for language immersion students are neutral. They are above the threshold below which bilingualism results in negative effects. The security of status of their L1, together with their parents' interest in their learning the L2 and the intensity of the school's commitment to the L2, with the addition of the general interest in language and familiarity with the kind of language used in cognitive-academic settings – all these things combine to eliminate any negative effects of bilingualism for the prototypic immersion student in Canada, according to Cummins (1976, 1979, and others).

The bilingualism developed under school immersion conditions may not be stable. Bruck, Lambert and Tucker (1974) reported that performance in French reading in the seventh grade for middle-class immersion children showed a marked decrease from the sixth-grade level. In the sixth grade the programme was altered to reduce the amount of instruction in French from nearly all of the time to about half of the time, and the French reading decrement seemed to be the result. Also, results of immersion programmes, even for middle-class children, may not always avoid negative results. Cowan and Sarmed (1976) found that children in English immersion programmes in Iran do not read either language as well as their monolingual peers at any grade. Cowan attributes the difference from the Canadian immersion results to the fact that English and Persian are more different from each other in structure and in orthography than are English and French, so that the cognitive sets created by English and Persian interfere with each other more, and also to some possible differences in subject group characteristics.

What happens to children in school language immersion programmes whose characteristics do not fit the prototype of those who successfully pass the lower threshold? Do all lower-class children show the negative consequences seen in the Finnish case? Even more pertinent to present concerns, how do children with below-average academic ability and children with learning disabilities fare in immersion programmes?

Genesee (1983) has reviewed research on these issues. According to him the suitability of immersion school programmes for lower-class children is still uncertain. Very little work has been done on 'hard-core' inner-city areas, but immersion programmes for more traditional working-class groups in the Montreal area have shown results which are, at least, not clearly negative. Several studies (Bruck, Tucker and Jakimik, 1975; Cziko, 1975; Tucker, Lambert and D'Anglejan, 1972) have found that in most cases these immersion pupils scored as well as the English control pupils in English language tests, and that they were not having special difficulty in mathematics. In French their listening comprehension was as good as French control students although more deficit was evident in other aspects of French. Genesee advocates caution concerning the suitability of immersion programmes for minority language children, and the need for more studies. He emphasises that the success of the Canadian programmes was probably closely related to the following factors: the use of the child's native language to teach curriculum material; an initial period during which the students are permitted to use their native language with one another and the teacher, even though the teacher speaks exclusively in the second language; an emphasis on the child's communicative use of the second language and not on correct grammatical usage; and a desire by the students, their parents and teachers to maintain development of the children's native language. It should be stressed also that these children's enrolment in the programme was approved and accepted by their parents, unlike in the Finnish case.

Genesee (1976, 1978) found that native English-speaking children of below average IQ scores (below 95) in the immersion programmes did not score significantly differently on English-language and mathematics tests than comparably low IQ monolingual English-speakers on these tests. Thus they appeared to be not differentially handicapped in their first-language development and academic achievement. In French, the L2 immersion language, these students scored lower than did average immersion students on reading and grammar tests, the tests which reflect the level of cognitive system understanding of language. However, on tests which assessed the basic interpersonal communication skills in French, i.e. speaking and listening comprehension, they scored as well as the average IQ immersion student. This outcome seems contrary to the notion of subtractive bilingualism. However, it is still not clear whether or not these students have experienced a language deficit from the immersion situation. If French reading and grammar accomplishment is low for them, it would seem that the academic content taught through French would suffer also, causing a cumulative cognitive deficit.

The research just discussed concerned immersion students who entered the immersion programme at kindergarten. Low IQ students who begin an immersion programme at a later age, around grade eleven, experience more clearly negative results. In this case low IQ is associated with low mastery of communication skills in French, i.e. low achievement in listening comprehension and in oral production (Genesee and Chaplin, 1976; Genesee and Stefanovic, 1976; Tucker, Hamayan and Genesee, 1976). It would appear that the late immersion programme is not beneficial for these students.

The findings for children with language or learning disabilities are mixed. In Bruck's research (1978, 1982), children of this type in early immersion programmes were matched with comparably disabled children in the regular English programme. Disability was determined by teachers and by a short diagnostic screening test devised by Bruck. The children had normal levels of intelligence by her measures. The results at the end of grade 3 indicated that it was taking the learning-disabled children in both programmes longer to attain basic literacy and academic skills than their non-disabled peers, but that the disabled children in the immersion programme had developed linguistic, cognitive and academic skills at a rate similar to that at which they would develop if placed in an all-English classroom. The disabled immersion students also showed progress in French learning to the point that they could cope with classroom instruction in French 'within the limits imposed by their disability'. Genesee concludes from Bruck's studies and from his own studies with low IQ students that these children 'do not experience additional disadvantage as a result of the immersion experience, and, to the contrary, they benefit from it in terms of improved second-language proficiency'.

In opposition to this, Trites (1981) contends that there is a distinct subgroup of children who cannot make satisfactory progress in early immersion programmes because they have a unique difficulty associated with a maturational lag in the development of temporal lobe regions of the brain. This is indicated by performance on a tactual performance task by students who had been having difficulties in the immersion programme. Genesee (1983) criticises Trites's conclusions on the grounds that his diagnosis is too specific, since these students did poorly on a whole range of tests in addition to the tactual performance test. He also criticises Trites's conclusion that the immersion programme is harmful to these children, since it is unknown whether these children would have experienced the same difficulties and lags in the regular monolingual programme.

Thus far we have discussed factors which determine whether consequences of immersion bilingualism will be negative or neutral, i.e. the lower threshold. Let us turn now to the factors which determine whether consequences of bilingualism will be neutral or positive -- the upper threshold.

As noted earlier, Cummins's conclusion is that the consequences of immersion bilingualism for normally intelligent middle-class children in an environment which values language and the particular aims of the bilingual school programme have primarily neutral effects on general cognition. The positive effects which have been found by research have been for children who have been bilingual from an early age and whose bilingualism developed in a natural setting, rather than from the school setting alone.

There is some evidence that for exceptionally intelligent students, even the immersion programmes as the source of bilingualism can have some positive effects on acquisition of convergent-type cognitive skill. Barik and Swain (1976) found that high French achievers in the immersion programme obtained significantly higher IQ scores and subtest scores (analogies and the following of verbal directions) than the low French achievers, even when scores were adjusted for initial IQ and age differences.

Turning now to those bilinguals who have been bilingual from an early age, and as the result of natural circumstances, two kinds of cognitive advantages have been found: (1) analytic skill; and (2) skill in perspective-taking or in switching frameworks.

Ben-Zeev (1976, 1977) studied two quite different groups of early bilinguals. The first were Hebrew-English bilinguals of ages 6-9 who developed their bilingualism in what would seem to be quite favourable circumstances. These children are from educated families who respect and encourage verbal behaviour. Both languages spoken by the children are highly valued in the communities in which they live. These bilinguals were compared to two control groups of similar ethno-religious and educational background, age and intelligence, one control group being monolingual English-speakers and the other monolingual Hebrew-speakers. The bilinguals were found to have superior analytic skills on linguistic tasks as well as, to some extent, non-linguistic tasks. On a test of ordinary syntax their performance did not differ from the monolingual control groups. However, they showed superior ability on a test which required them to treat a word of a sentence as if it were a desemanticised unit of a code system. This task involved ability to overcome word magic, and thus to separate the meaning of a word from its actual referent. It also involved the ability to substitute one part of speech for another, which involves understanding of language structure outside of its usual situational context. On non-verbal tests these bilinguals were better able to isolate from each other and name the two interacting dimensions of a matrix. On a test called 'verbal transformations', which involved illusions created by a continuously repeated nonsense syllable, the bilinguals thought they heard more different forms and changes, as if they were looking more intensely than the control groups for some way of interpreting the stimulus. On the Ravens Matrices Test, although these bilinguals were not different from controls in main score, they were better able to resist simply choosing the response item closest to the choice point instead of scanning the whole field of possible responses. At the same time, however, these bilinguals showed a clear vocabulary deficit on the Peabody Vocabulary Test.

Ianco-Worrall (1972) found for South African bilinguals whose bilingualism was developed in circumstances more or less comparable to the above that the bilinguals were more attuned to meaning relationships between words than to mere sound relationships, in comparison to their control group.

Cummins and Mulcahy (1978) found that those Ukranian-English bilinguals in Canada who had learned Ukranian at home, not just in the school immersion programme, were better able to analyse ambiguities in sentence structure than were either non-fluent bilinguals or monolingual controls, all groups being equated for IQ, social class, sex and age.

The other bilingual group studied by Ben-Zeev was quite different. They were Spanish-English bilinguals from poverty-level neighbourhoods of Chicago. The English grammar of these bilinguals was clearly inferior to their monolingual control group of similar ethnicity, IQ, social class, sex and age, although their sentences were equally complex in structure. The pattern they showed across a number of different tests can be interpreted as less a matter of analytic skill than of ability to switch points of view as required, – a sort of flexibility of perspective. In particular, they were especially responsive to feedback cues indicating the need to switch to a different point of view. The pattern could be characterised as a reactive mechanism developed to correct quickly mistakes made concerning which language was being spoken or of incorrect use of the language. It involved a readiness to switch away from an incorrect framework. These bilinguals manifested clearly lowered vocabulary scores relative to their control group, as did the Hebrew-English group.

One might ask why the children in the immersion programmes did not show more positive cognitive consequences such as these? The answer is probably related to the level of their mastery of the second language. According to Genesee (1978), in relation to native speakers of French, students who learn their French entirely through the French immersion programme are likely to score as well on tests that assess the ability to *decode* French: namely, on listening comprehension and reading comprehension. As for *productive* language skills – namely, speaking, or knowledge of discrete linguistic rules on a grammar test – the immersion students were judged good, but less than native-like. Thus it seems that their passive knowledge of French is better than their active usage.

Bruck, Lambert and Tucker (1976) found that in oral telling of a silent film story to someone who had not seen the film, the immersion students recounted the same amount and kinds of information in French as did the native French. Similarly, immersion students are given high subjective ratings for communicative competence in face-to-face conversations. Genesee (1983) notes, however, that in face-to-face situations the grammar usage of these bilinguals is not native-like. They simplify verb use and make many types of errors. He suggests that this apparent facility in second-language communicative competence might reflect the greater availability of non-linguistic cues in the types of communicative interactions that have been used for assessment. In other words, these bilinguals might be relying upon situational context rather than more strictly linguistic processing, meaning that their competence is relatively superficial.

The students themselves often expressed personal reservations about their interpersonal communication skills. They perceive a difference between the type of French they learn and use in school and that needed for informal peer situations (Genesee, 1978).

Perhaps the notion of communicative competence, as it has been measured, is too lax and undefined. Psychologists of child language have often cautioned (e.g. Hakes, 1982; Hickman, 1982) that language behaviour that appears to be decontextualised may actually be processed at a much lower level. Another problem is that the language behaviour of these immersion bilinguals does not seem to fit neatly into a division Cummins (1976) made between the basic communicative competence level of language and the kind of analytic understanding necessary for language usage in an academic context. Theoretically, cognitive-academic competence should include high skill in reading which results from high levels of structure mastery. This would seem to entail high mastery of syntax. Yet these bilinguals are said to have reading skill in their L2 which is as high as that of native speakers, but without the mastery of syntax which this would seem to entail. Another source of evidence which shows the advanced immersion bilinguals performing as well as native French speakers is a study by Cziko (1975). This showed that seventh-grade immersion students benefitted from reading a meaningful text as compared to a meaningless text as much as did native speakers, and that among the meaningless texts, they benefitted to the same degree as the natives from texts that retained expected order of parts of speech and typical agreement rules between nouns and verbs. However, although Cziko refers to the latter type of text as syntactically correct, as compared to a text with words thrown together totally at random, this is really only one level of syntax. The study did not attempt to emphasise syntactic structures in which the contrast between French and English is especially strong. Thus we cannot draw the general conclusion that immersion students have mastered the syntax involved in reading.

The measure used in the above study was speed of reading. Concerning speed, recent papers (Daitchman, 1976; Favreau, Komoda and Segalowitz, 1980) found that adult bilinguals who are apparently more highly skilled and experienced in their second language than the immersion subjects, as determined by the fact that their vocabulary and syntax mastery of L2 is high, read more slowly in their second language than their first. Favreau and Segalowitz (1982) went on to show that bilinguals who read more slowly in their second language also selected a slower rate of delivery for incoming auditory information in that language. This means that they comprehend that information more slowly too. There is also evidence in this study that the theoretical distinction between 'subtractive' and 'additive' bilingualism cannot be made as sharply as in the original conceptualisation, at least not at high levels of mastery. Those bilinguals who were most balanced in skill between their two languages, in that their speed in both languages was more nearly equal, also were slower in both languages than the other type of bilingual. Thus, in their mastery equivalency these bilinguals have an 'additive' type of bilingualism, but in their speed of comprehension, their skill is to some extent 'subtractive'. Of course, this notion of 'subtractiveness' is relatively mild compared to the serious cognitive effects of the subtractive situation hypothesised by Lambert. These bilinguals have, after all, achieved a very high level of bilingualism.

Similarly to the 'additive-subtractive' distinction, the distinction between 'basic communicative competence' vs. 'cognitive-academic' language competence is another distinction that is very useful but that can benefit from elaboration and qualification, because the line cannot be drawn as sharply as it originally may have seemed. It may be that there is a limit to the 'cognitive-academic' level of language which can be achieved through a school learning situation. It may be that the highest levels of language achievement may have to grow directly out of the contextually supported situations in which speech is first learned. The immersion bilinguals, having missed these early stages of childhood speech in L2, perhaps cannot develop the structure of their language on the decontextualised level to the extent that a native speaker potentially can. This is not to denigrate immersion programmes, for they clearly have been very successful at what they set out to do. It is merely to say that there may be upper limits to language that develops outside of the usual course of child development, with its heavy backing of situational support, in which the closeness of speech to action and to perception makes meaning eminently obvious.

Cummins's distinction between 'basic communicative competence' and 'cognitive-academic' language competence is based on the theories of Bruner (1966) and of Olson (1977) concerning the influence of schooling, and especially of reading and writing. These authors see informal face-to-face conversation as inexplicit and heavily dependent on context for interpretation, so that language here is not being employed as an independent system. Schooling, in contrast, demands that the child talk about things outside of the immediate context, and since it is not therefore so obvious what is being talked about, the speaker must be more explicit. The need to be explicit forces the speaker to be self-conscious of his language and to use it as an independent system. Even more than speech in a school context, reading demands decontextualisation and explicitness. Writing demands these to an even greater degree of consciousness.

These ideas are very important for understanding linguistic and cognitive development. Greenfield (1966) has shown that even a small amount of schooling in very modest bush schools for African tribal children leads to clear increases in conversation performance on Piagetian tests, when these children are compared to their tribal peers who have had no schooling because of the lack of facilities or similar reasons. However, although it may be true that talk in school and most written language in school is more explicit than informal talk, and that it is generally less related to the immediate context, explicitness is only one of the ways in which language can act as a tool to advance cognitive development. Another way is to serve as a taking-off point for inference-making and perspective-taking. In this regard, written speech is the means for the highest development of these skills, but it is not the exclusive medium for development.

Informal conversation can require these skills also. There are a variety of kinds of informal conversation, some of which require no more than the basic level of communication Cummins discusses, and some of which require repeated on-the-spot calculation on the part of each participant concerning the level of familiarity of the interlocutor with each successive topic, and quick estimations of the interlocutor's ability to infer meaning from minimal cues. Here the speaker constantly gauges and regauges the perspective of his interlocutor.

Prince (1981) closely examined an informal narrative, taken without the knowledge of the speaker. The speaker was a middle-aged, middle-class, educated woman, whose narrative concerned a domestic accident that happened on the way to a luncheon gathering. Prince showed how the speaker manipulated the assumed familiarity level of the hearer, so that use of the hearer's assumed frame of reference could allow an impressive amount of information to be conveyed which was neither explicit nor present in the context. Prince then showed how a formal text, written for professional linguists, requires a far greater amount of meta-linguistic inferencing on the part of the receiver of the text. She says:

> Contra Olson, where it is claimed that written language is explicit whereas oral language leaves much out, the analyses presented here suggest that just the opposite is the case: The comprehension of formal, literary discourse depends a great deal more on inference, quantitatively and qualitatively, than the processing of informal colloquial discourse.

Actually, the characterisation of speech and writing in grade school as explicit is probably a good characterisation, and in this sense, Bruner and Olson are correct in their description of formal school speech. But the most demanding types of language-processing, particularly in written form, as in great literature, require high inferencing skill and the ability to take various successive and simultaneous perspectives. As for elementary school speech and writing, in so far as it is decontextualised it does probably tend to stimulate analysis, but it does not always require much perspective-taking. The very explicitness partially eliminates the need for perspective-taking. In fact, this type of speech must be considered as constituting a domain of its own. As such, it has its own kind of predictability and its own highly probable forms. It is even possible that much of this type of speech and writing can be understood by middle-class students, including immersion bilinguals, even without very deep mastery or consciousness of the real discourse structure of the particular language. The general ability to deal with decontextualised situations which comes with being middle-class, together with the relative syntactic predictability of school-type speech and writing, may be sufficient.

It may be that the high-level inference-making and perspective-taking that is demanded by the higher forms of reading and writing, when they are mastered, are the outcome and later development of an earlier stage in middle-class life in which experience is gained in the kind of inference-packed conversations described by Prince.

In general, how can the language learner get from the deeply contextualised speech characteristic of every individual's early childhood to the highest level? The link may be Prince's type of decontextualised informal conversation. It may be that if the child lacks the successive experiences of working through strict contextualisation of language and later relative decontextualisation in conversational contexts, he may never gain the skill to reach the highest stages of reading and writing. The child who learns both languages early has this opportunity available to him, if he lives in the kind of environment where considerable inferencing is used in informal speech. In deprived environments such experience is less available, even to monolinguals, because the level of interaction remains relatively more concrete. Individuals who learn their second language through immersion prorgrammes in school, even if middle class, and who do not have informal conversational experience in the second language, may have limitations in the level of higher literacy they can achieve, although they are able to achieve much.

This must be qualified by the finding of Genesee, Tucker and Lambert (1975) that Canadian immersion students did better than monolingual controls on an interpersonal communication task that required sensitivity to the listener's needs. The question is the depth of this effect, and whether the bilinguals' limitations in syntactic knowledge allow them to give full expression to such sensitivity in ongoing speech. More work remains to be done.

Early Language: The Importance of Contextual Support and of Early Structure upon Later Structure

This concerns how language develops out of the immediate situational context into its later structure, in the mind of the individual. In later stages of language knowledge, in normal individuals' past childhood, there is usually still strong reliance on context for language interpretation and production, but the individual contributes, as well, perspectives from memories which arise in the flow of discourse, and which modify the stimuli coming in from the immediate situation. The memories can concern the topic, the listener, etc. Such influences affect rhetorical style, discourse structure and syntax. For all these influences to result in speech behaviour that communicates to the listener, the speaker must have sufficient control to combine them into a meaningful adaptive linguistic flow. This kind of skill is clearly adaptive for any language situation, whether monolingual or bilingual. For the bilingual, such flexible control over the set of perspectives being negotiated in ongoing speech may be especially important.

When a child cannot develop this kind of flexibility, either because of retardation or because of a language disability, the child can benefit from continuing reliance on the immediate external action situation for support and for disambiguation. This may be especially important for bilingual children with language disability.

The following evidence supports the essentiality of context support for language meaning in the earliest language period, and outlines the early stages of syntactic knowledge, i.e. of rising above context.

In the earliest sentences spoken by adult to child, the syntax of the sentence is not necessary to the understanding of the sentence. In English, for example, Slobin and Bever (1983) found that in almost every utterance involving two nouns and a verb, the agent of the action was animate and the object of the action inanimate. This entails that only one of the nouns could plausibly be the agent. The meaning is completely predictable from the context.

At age three to four a child begins to notice the basic marking devices of his language (Slobin and Bever, 1983). These may consist primarily of noun or verb inflections or primarily of word order, or the particular language may require some combination of these devices. In English the relation between agent and object of the sentence is signalled very strongly by agent-object word order and by the presence of the verb between agent noun and object noun. What the child learns at this age is not only the prototypic word order, but also the probability and reliability of this order. For example, the child learning Italian learns the prototypic word order of Italian. This order is the same as for English but is much less reliable, since in Italian other devices interact with order. The Italian child learns to rely more on the relative animacy of the referents of the two candidate nouns in the sentence to determine which represents the agent than on word order, and judges the more animate of the two nouns to be the agent (Bates and MacWhinney, 1982).

Syntax addressed to the child usually is much simplified, and even when it is not, the child will either misinterpret a more complex form like the passive as another example of the simple construction, or will not interpret it at all (Bever, 1970; Slobin and Bever, 1983; Strohner and Nelson, 1974).

The child of about this age, by learning how his language represents the basic action relations within its particular syntax, has learned two things crucial to the development of the more complex syntax system which develops later, and, very likely, crucial also to the ability to differentiate between two languages. These things are: (1) which of four competing functions are the most important for the structure of his language; and (2) what aspects intrinsic to the relation of a referent to its environment are directly coded into the lexical verbs of the particular language?

The functions which compete for starting position in the structure of language sentences are: the agent, the given, the focus and the perspective (MacWhinney, 1977). In English, for example, the very high probability that agent will be coded into initial sentence position, whether agent was given by previous context or not, demonstrates that relationships of given vs. new are unimportant in English, relative to some other language. The child of age 3-4 learns that English sentences begin with agent reference. At this point the child is incapable of coding changes in perspective or focus, so the prototype of initial agent reference is especially strong.

In contrast to English, in Spanish both givenness and agency are more in competition for first position. The child must learn to judge between them in a particular case by taking into consideration other characteristics of the context. At first this is only the external situational context. Much later the intralingual sentence context, the way one sentence follows another, and refers back to another, becomes primary. In Russian the given-new distinction is dominant in determining the starting point of the sentence, so the child learns to determine agency by some means other than initial position – in this case by inflectional marking (Slobin and Bever, 1983).

This kind of learning is extremely important to language development because it determines the child's expectations at the beginning of every sentence. Language comprehension and ease of reading are influenced by the ability to predict structure (Smith, F. 1973).

Bates and MacWhinney (1982) did a preliminary study of highly-educated adult bilinguals who became bilingual past early childhood. They have lived for many years in the US, their adopted country, and some write professionally in their adopted language. It was found that most of these bilinguals still use their native language structure rather than English structure as the model for deciding which noun, in various orderings of two English nouns and a verb, represents the agent. This may be related to Newport's finding (1982) that deaf adults who did not learn sign language until later childhood used 'frozen signs', which lacked many of the grammatical characteristics by which native signers integrate individual words into the structure of the sentence.

The second function which appears to be learned early is the relation of the meaning of the lexical verb of the sentence to basic syntax. According to Talmy (1984), different languages express, along with the basic motion meaning of the verb, particular kinds of auxiliary notions within the verb itself. For example, English, along with some other Indo-European languages and Chinese, tends to express both the notion of cause and the notion of manner on the verb itself. In contrast, Spanish must express these notions by auxiliary means, outside of the verb. On the other hand, Spanish and some other languages tend to express the notion of path on the verb itself. For still another contrast, various Indian languages express the notion of shape and texture of the object of the verb on the verb itself. For example: English motion + manner: I *rolled* the ball into the box, i.e. I moved the ball into the box by means of rolling it. English motion + cause: The napkin *blew* off the table, i.e. The napkin moved off the table from the wind's blowing on it. Spanish motion + path: Pablo estaba escuchando esa cancion, i.e. Paul was *listening to* that song.

The tendencies for linguistic functioning which are built into the child from early experience with language at this stage are better thought of not as rote learning but as a set of expectations. These comprise a beginning structure upon which later language structure is built. The later and more complex structure is a more canalised development from the earlier structure and it depends upon the earlier structure.

Let us take the early learning of word order in English, for example. The early learning of agent-action-object prototypic order predisposes the English-speaker away from a type of later construction called 'clause union', common in Romance and other languages. In this construction, two verbs are joined into one and the resulting sentence represents one agent causing another to act. Since there cannot be more than one person in agent role in a given clause, the second agent must assume some other case role in the sentence, which is usually indirect object or object of a 'by' clause, as in the following French example:

Jean les fera acheter à Marie.
Jean them will make to buy to Marie.
(Jean will have Marie buy them.)

English-speakers find this difficult because it violates the great consistency of agent in initial position in English and perhaps also because of the high transitivity of the verb in English, which assumes cause within itself so readily. The point is that the biases in a language which begin to be understood by the child in the third or fourth year make it difficult for him to learn at a later time structures of another language built upon a different set of biases. Even if they show considerable fluency in the second language, there is still a certain superficiality, usually, because of the clash with initial structural bias.

Another example of the effect of early structure bias in L1 on L2 is seen in the grammatical judgements of Mexican-Americans, who accept some forms in Spanish which are clearly influenced by English, but who would usually not accept the sentence:

Traeme el libro sobre la cama.
(Bring me the book on the bed.)

(Lantolf, 1980). In Spanish the feeling is that the path vector is within the verb ('bring toward'), and that no other path vector (e.g. *sobre* la cama) is needed in the same clause.

A language also brings with it its own ways of changing perspective. In the early years it is a matter of simple changes of stance, as for statements v. questions v. exclamations, etc.; changes in aspect appear quite early, and later come distinctions between hypothetical v. real. The early, gross types of changes are represented in every language's syntax, but as changes become more subtle, the grammars of different languages vary greatly in which perspective changes are incorporated into the grammatical system and which not. As each language becomes more canalised, it becomes increasingly difficult to negotiate between two language systems, because of the perspectival and other syntactic differences. What is required is either a high level of metalinguistic skill to maintain the interaction between the language structures while adhering to the rules of each, or else some means to seal off the languages from contact with each other.

Very young children, when faced with the demand to learn two languages, will try the sealing-off method, even at that early stage when the structures are less canalised. Thus the child will resist by refusing to speak the language which he perceives to be less valued, if such an option is available (Itoh and Hatch, 1978). When this option is not available, because both languages are highly valued and necessary in his environment, the child will tend to become especially adept at reading clues which allow him to judge which language is appropriate in which context. The cues concern proper domain or characteristics of the interlocutor (Fantini, 1978). This is probably why the child can function without disabling mutual interference between his languages (Lindholm and Padilla, 1978).

The cues which young bilingual children use to separate their languages are of an obvious type. Older skilled bilinguals can use more subtle cues, both from the outside and from inner feelings and associations. When speaking to another bilingual with similar background to his, he can switch languages in mid-sentence. He does this either to create a desired rhetorical effect, or because the immediate subject being discussed in language A at that point brings in associations to events, persons, etc. in language B, or for other reasons. He can switch languages flexibly without violating the rules of either language (Pfaff, 1979; Poplack, 1982).

The young child in a bilingual environment has not internalised the two languages as systems sufficiently to switch in a very skilled manner. He needs the framework provided by the external situational context much more. The external situation proper to each language, respectively, ensconces him within it while he is in that frame, and few bridges are built. This minimises the possibilities for interference between the two languages in early childhood.

Problems can arise as the bilingual gets into the middle school years, into what approximates Piaget's concrete-operational stage of thought. He becomes more capable of bringing different contexts into relationship with each other. He also encounters more circumstances in which it is uncertain which language is to be used. The child may develop certain mechanisms to counteract the problem, which have already been mentioned. These are: (1) a sort of vigilance developed to forestall the need for reorientation – if one can learn the cues for preventing being taken by surprise, one avoids the need to react to it; and (2) the development of ability to switch presuppositional frameworks quickly, once interference has indeed occurred.

As for the first factor, we have already discussed how important it is to the child to have a decipherable situation in the environment as the basis for language-learning. In the case noted above the child seeks to maximise decipherability by becoming sensitive to cues such as the sound of the language, the look or accent of interlocutor, the location, the subject matter, etc. Fantini (1978) has described how sensitive a bilingual child can be to cues of this sort, and how he may refuse to speak a language with an individual who seems to him inappropriate for that language framework. The child attempts to maximise predictability by attending to factors associated with differentiating the two respective language contexts.

To summarise: at the lower levels of language experience and accomplishment high context dependence minimises interference. When faced with interference, the child tries to simplify his environment by ignoring one of the languages. At a higher level, he develops special discrimination skill. At a still higher level of skill, he internalises each of the language structures, to some extent, so that he need not rely on the external situation for discrimination purposes. In this case he may achieve an unusual level of metalinguistic understanding, both in terms of understanding of grammatical structure and of perspective-taking.

Language-disabled Bilinguals

Consider now language-disabled children whose environment challenges them from an early age to become bilingual. How does their deficit influence their bilingualism, and how does the challenge influence their cognitive development? There is not much direct evidence, but there is enough related evidence to draw hypotheses which require further research. There is considerable evidence that language-disabled children (as defined, usually, by problems with reading together with relatively normal IQ) are deficient in processing the syntax of their language (see review by Vellutino, 1980).

There is also evidence that language-disabled children have difficulty in adjusting the form of their speech appropriately to the social perspective of their interlocutors. Donahue (1981) found that such children have difficulty using the terminology available to them to use persuasive rhetoric appropriate to the perspective of the person whose opinion they are trying to influence.

The Problem of Distinguishing Incomplete Bilingualism from Language Disability

Earlier in this chapter we discussed the problem of separating the diagnosis of language disability from low IQ and from low vocabulary. There are also other problems of diagnosis of language disability in relation to bilingualism.

It is not uncommon for each language code of a bilingual to be specialised to a particular set of domains, so that neither code develops the full stylistic variation which it would have if the person were monolingual. For some individuals, for example, some groups of Mexican-Americans, it is difficult to change domains of speech without code-switching. It is interesting that grammatical distinctions in Spanish might be very well maintained for a particular domain. Lavendera (1981) found that Spanish aspectual distinctions in such a group of bilinguals are maintained very well for the domain of narratives in the past, which these speakers associate with the Spanish linguo-cultural framework, but that when they talk of events in the present and outside of the narrative frame, their use of Spanish aspect becomes blurred and contaminated by transfer from the simpler English system.

Here, then, is another way that context is important to language, overriding any sense of perfect syntactic consistency. In this case we are speaking not of immediate situational context, because past narratives are far from dependent upon immediate context, and, in fact, require considerable ability to internalise and abstract from immediacy, but it is context nevertheless.

In testing children for possible language disability, care should be taken to see that a variety of context domains are sampled, since consistent use of syntactic rules differs from one domain to another.

Another phenomenon which can lead to misdiagnosis is the phenomenon called 'syntactic calquing' by Stewart (1982), which accompanies imperfect bilingualism. Here the speaker routinely applies the structure of his first language to his second language. The form that this syntactic translation takes may appear to be an ordinary sentence of L2, and not at all ungrammatical, although actually in the mind of the speaker it represents a different structure, one directly based on a similar form in L1. Stewart shows this effect operating for Black English, and Gumperz (1982) gives numerous examples of how Indian speakers of fluent English may appear to their interlocutors to be saying something either stupid or quite insensitive, when what they are intending to say is something very different. For further discussion on this point the reader is directed to Chapter 4, and the notion of covert and overt errors. It would be wise for those who are responsible for determining language disability to know the child's native language and to be able to use some imagination concerning the possible appearance of such subtle syntactic mistranslations. Fluent but incomplete bilingualism may sometimes look like language disability.

In conclusion, regarding the relationship of bilingualism and cognition, the findings in the literature are not difficult to outline. Negative effects of bilingualism on school learning tend to appear for underprivileged immigrant sectors of the population, though even for underprivileged immigrant children, when their bilingualism is not totally dependent upon the school for its existence, so that both languages are used out of school as well, the bilingualism can create a certain reactive flexibility of perspective, which can be regarded as a positive effect. Neutral effects arise with middle-class immersion programmes such as those in Canada in which speakers of the dominant language voluntarily choose immersion in the language of the non-dominant culture in their school experience. Positive effects of bilingualism involve metalinguistic types of understanding, such as sentence ambiguity, ability to mark and substitute the basic word units of a sentence, as well as the basic units of a non-verbal matrix system; and flexibility in reorganising, or reclassifying the units of a non-verbal system according to different points of view. This is in addition to the less tangible and less quantifiable advantages of having potential access to two or more linguistic-cultural communities. However, sorting out the factors behind these findings is much more difficult. Earlier opinions that there was a direct causal relationship between being bilingual (which was simplistically defined as using two languages without consideration of which ones, when or how) and cognitive and emotional development have been demonstrated to be too simple. This chapter has suggested some of the additional factors, both internal and external to the individual, that need to be considered in a more realistic appraisal of the interaction between bilingualism and cognition that determine the above variations in findings. Differences derive as much from broader social factors which determine timing, incentive and opportunity and the nature of the child's access to the languages involved as they do from features inherent in the language concerned and from the child's general and (language) specific development. The proper assessment of a (potentially) bilingual individual and effective remedial intervention must consider all these factors in gaining an accurate diagnostic and prognostic picture. Some of the difficulties in this task were touched upon, but are taken up in more detail in the chapters more directly dealing with the issues involved.

4 LANGUAGE PROBLEMS AND BILINGUAL CHILDREN

Niklas Miller

Defining the Problem: Normal Variation

The notion of 'problem' is a highly subjective area. The word *and* is used in the title of this chapter advisedly, to imply that there exists a body of utterances spoken or written by particular individuals or groups of people, which might result in the person using them being classed as having a language problem. However, the assignment of this label is in general not an objective exercise. While there may be utterances at either end of the 'normal'-'disordered' scale of language development and usage that could relatively incontrovertibly be agreed on as betraying the presence or absence of a language problem, in the considerable grey middleground between these extremes whole areas of usage are to be found where decisions on whether or not the sample is indicative of an underlying problem depend on many factors. It is true that there are aspects of language acquisition and execution which would permit one to talk of the language problems of bilingual children, but by and large judgements are made according to many criteria, very few of which are linked immediately to any objectively quantifiable inherent property of language as a system independent of the context in which it is employed. 'Problem' in this view is context-sensitive. What in one instance is branded a problem will be taken as normal in another place, with another person or at another time. Thus it is perhaps more honest to study initially under what circumstances the term 'problem' becomes ascribed to particular usages or persons, rather than the construction of some parameter(s) whereby the linguistic analysis of the phonological or syntactic details will set what must be considered with our present state of knowledge, quantification and attitudes, only a pseudo-objective score on a scale normal-to-problem for a particular corpus of data. The problem might be as much in the ear of the listener as in the mouth of the speaker. Hence it is preferred to speak here of language 'problems' *and* under what conditions bilingual children might be described as experiencing them, as opposed to the inference in the use of *of*, that problems emanate from the individual in the nature of a contagious virus.

Value judgements about language made on the basis of social-cultural prejudices represent a major area of 'problem' finding. Past feelings on correctness and error (since problem is equated by many with someone else's 'difficulty' in using their form, the 'correct' form, irrespective of whether the speaker set out to produce it in the first place or not) and the influence of this on attitudes to bilinguals' language was mentioned in Chapter 1. Trudgill (1975) has discussed the persisting effects of these attitudes in relation to monolingual children's language variation, while V.K. Edwards (1979) has conducted a similar discussion in relation to the supposed language problems of West Indian children, a subject also touched upon in HMSO (1981), and J. Edwards (1979) has examined the role of expectations and value judgements about non-standard usage in the field of language and disadvantage. The discussion concerning the 'difference' versus 'deficit' debate in language development and use is amply covered in these works, and although the points made are highly relevant to the present topic, economy of space unfortunately precludes more detailed analysis here. Suffice it to say that in seeking to find whether a bilingual child has a language problem or is cognitively retarded, one must consider whether a genuine difficulty in expressing meanings linguistically does exist, or whether his/her utterances represent simply a different way of saying something, in which case they do not constitute a cognitive or developmental deficit, and the assignment of a label would be a statement on social grounds.

Judgements may relate to variation in syntactic-morphological realisation ('I didn't never went there' v. 'I didn't ever go there'), appropriateness and accuracy of lexical choice (my moggy v. cat ran away; 'He likes to eat sweetness', instead of sweets; 'Sunday I visited my babka', rather than grandmother) or the associations certain accents might have in a particular community. See for instance J. Edwards (1977) for a monolingual Irish example, or Ryan, Carranza and Moffie (1977) for reactions of English-speaking students to varying degrees of accentedness in Spanish-English bilinguals' reading. Some listeners are easily blinded (or deafened?) to sound underlying expressive abilities by their subjective impressions formed on the basis of surface differences.

Variation associated with the bilingual context does not constitute the sole source of variation for bilingual children. There are also sources which operate equally for the bilingual and monolingual child. Wells (1979) discusses age, sex, intelligence and personality, caretaker-child interaction and others. In L1 acquisition the caretaker's input and reactions can shape the child's language style and content at different stages. Variations cross-culturally in who acts as caretaker (grandparent, elder siblings, communal child-minders) and the patterns of usage this might produce is an area for research both in child language variation and in its possible relevance in remediation with language-disordered children.

Sociolinguistically determined variation is not the only natural source of differences in child language. Another source of mistaken error/problem assignment, particularly from those unfamiliar with the normal course of language development, or who have over-optimistic expectations regarding its rate, is branding as problems utterances that may not be identical to the adult language accepted forms, but which may nevertheless be an acceptable form according to the processes in the emerging grammar of the child. Children do not wake up one morning suddenly speaking like adults any more than they wake up one day and dribble a ball around a football pitch. Neither do they progress by adding chunks of the adult language together like a jigsaw. Rather, language development in terms of approximation to the adult system is a gradual process taking place over a period of several years, during which time the child's own grammatical rules will be constantly modified. At any one stage there will be utterances produced which may not comply with adult 'rules' but which must be considered correct within the child's system. The same must be said for bilingual children. They also, do not wake up one morning completely fluent in their second (or first) language but proceed through recognisable stages, as was discussed in Chapter 2. One of the major exercises in assessing language is to differentiate between normal developmental patterns and genuine problems outside of generally recognised stages of acquisition.

Research into child language development over the past two decades has uncovered the remarkable similarities that pertain in the nature of the learning process not only from one child to another within the same language community (Brown, 1973; P. de Villiers and J. de Villiers, 1979) but also, remarkably, across different languages (Slobin, 1970; Bowerman, 1973). These similarities have been exploited in constructing assessment materials (Crystal, Fletcher and Garman, 1976; Lee, 1974) which analyse a corpus of a child's language with reference to descriptions of stages of development – one word, holophrastic stage, two-word utterances, emergence of number-marking, aspect-marking and so on.

The majority of language acquisition studies concentrate on the early years of development. It must not, however, be forgotten that language development is taking place before the child utters his first 'words' and far from being completed by the age of three years, as was at one time the contention, children continue to develop language and experience normal problems well after this age – see in this respect Karmiloff-Smith (1979), Lapointe (1976), and Wiig (1976).

The search for universals in the acquisition process should not, however, blind one to the fact that despite a strong degree of cross-cultural uniformity in the order of acquisition of linguistic features there are many children who do not conform to the expected processes and yet still need not be classed as suffering language problems. The end goal for most children is adult competency in communication, but they do not apparently all have to follow the same road.

A closer examination of the child's lexical development illustrates this point. The child's vocabulary does not commence as a miniature version of the adult's with development simply by accretion of new words. The verbal labels the child employs may resemble certain adult words, but usage is not necessarily the same. Thus *doggy* (or the child's various phonological realisations of this) might refer not (only) to the four-legged furry animal that says woof, but any animal, the person who takes the dog for a walk and/or the dog's lead. Further, this single lable *dog* may function as both statement (that's a dog), question (where's the dog; is that a dog) and command (give me the dog). Grieve and Hoogenraad (1976, 1979), studying children's early words, point to the many communicative functions which first words fulfil beyond direct labelling, the variations which occur in what a lexical item refers to and children's uncertainty about the meaning of particular words. They also mention the uncertainties in the pronunciation of words. This includes not only variation attributable to the child's developing phonological system, but also idiosyncratic versions. Crystal (1981) characterises the child's semantic mismatches broadly in terms of under-extension (p. 178, *bus* being used solely for red buses), over-extension (as in the doggy example above) and no overlap, when *bird* might be used for *cake.*

Difficulties involving pronunciation may persist into adulthood. Many grown-ups frequently mispronounce words like statistics or certificate. One strategy children use when confronted with unmanageable words is to reinterpret them in terms of words familiar to them. Aitchison (1972) provides many examples of mini-malapropisms and from the author's own data could be cited the use by a normal monolingual eight-year-old of *biscuetti* for *spaghetti*, or a *Dora rabbit* for *angora rabbit*. These examples are not absent from adult language, again, from own data, come *shallots* for *culottes*, *sizzling* for *soliciting* and *national* for *maximum*.

Further adult 'errors' which are found in child language are the attachment of the wrong understanding or expression to a word, by confusion with either a similar sounding or a similar structured word – e.g. specific-pacific; irritating-irritable; disinterested-uninterested.

Nelson (1975) has noted another area of developmental variation. The data she presented show how some children possess a large lexicon before they begin to combine words into two- or three-word utterances, while others produce multi-word utterances almost from the start. Qualitative differences in the nature of the lexicon disclosed how some children had words referring predominantly to things and actions, while others had a greater percentage that expressed desires or could influence others.

Many children typically display errors in certain lexico-grammatical contexts. The extensive literature on the apparent difficulties in the use of *more* and *less* has been discussed by Grieve (1981) and other antonymical pairs by M. Richards (1979). *Tell* versus *ask* in such sentences as *Ask/Tell Jan what to give his mummy* is a commonly reported difficulty up to certain levels of development. Cromer (1970) highlighted the problems of comprehension faced by some children with sentences like *the wolf is happy to bite* v. *the wolf is tasty to bite*.

Developmental 'errors' also arise with syntax and morphology. A frequent one is the misunderstanding of the passive construction *the dog was chased by Liam* in terms of the agent-action-object word order of active declarative structures, leading to the false impression that the dog was doing the chasing. Bloom, Lightbown and Hood (1975) give examples of normal variation in pronominal and nominal acquisition.

Clearly the scope for such 'errors' arising in the bilingual situation is considerable. Aside from the types of normal variation noted previously, there are the added factors occurring associated with the code-switching for topic, setting or interpersonal reasons described in Chapter 2. For instance, in the lexical field it frequently happens that children know a word for something in one of their languages, but not in the other. In the normal child this might provoke the use of gesture, using the word from the other language or circumlocution. The child with difficulties often reacts with silence. Nelson-Burgess and Meyerson's (1975) MIRA represents an attempt at assessing a child's overall lexical development.

The rates at which these developments take place is also a source of intersubject variation. Although the onset of the first words is taken to be between twelve and eighteen months (leaving aside the question of what is to count as a first word) earlier and later onset still within normal limits does occur. See for instance, Prather, Hedrick and Kern (1975) and the acquisition of speech sounds. Later development may show even greater discrepancies between earliest and latest probable times of appearance of features. Some aspects of language usage may in fact never be acquired by some people, and certain features of acquisition and performance may show defects right into adulthood. The recognition and understanding of the roots of variation in normal language is crucial in striving to appreciate non-normal language, which after all is only another form of variation.

Dulay, Hernández-Chávez and Burt (1978), reviewing the systematic nature of learning errors in L1 and L2, in their conclusions considered that the 'creative errors' in L2 learning reflected in kind the slips in L1 acquisition. To this extent a knowledge of L1 acquisition literature would be fruitful in studying L2 learners' language, but only in as far as it reflected the workings of the postulated common (to L1, L2) language acquisition device. On top of it one must consider the different sociocultural context of learning and usage. The genesis of errors in L2 comprehension and production still arouses some controversy, however, and the background to the arguments is outlined later in this chapter.

Defining the Problem: Non-normal Variation

What is a language disorder? The majority of children have a fair command of (first) language in a relatively short time, without requiring formal instruction. There are, however, other children whose development is overall far slower than the normally accepted limits or who may exhibit a pattern of acquisition not typical of normal children, requiring formal intervention to bring their language into line with their normal peers and who in some cases may never complete the language acquisition process beyond a rudimentary level. The terminology used in the literature to label such children is highly varied, at times controversial, and includes language impaired, linguistically deficient, language deviant, aphasic and other.

It is possible to view such disorders from several angles, according to one's purpose and role. This may vary from the speech and language clinician looking at the pre-spoken language of the nine-month-old baby, to the educational psychologist assessing the four-year-old for school placement or the remedial teacher coping with the speaking and reading problems of a child in class.

Two of the main perspectives that might influence these people's views are what Bloom and Lahey (1978, p. 305) have termed the categorical and specific abilities orientations versus a linguistic orientation. Crystal (1980, p. 17) has labelled this same division medical versus behavioural model. These are not the sole ways of looking at language disorder – see Crystal (1980, p. 49) – but are currently the most widespread.

Broadly speaking the medical model derives from a nosological approach to language disorders, giving weight in diagnosis and remediation to aetiological factors, e.g. mental retardation, neurological, emotional and audiological origins. Specific abilities classifications order impaired children in relation to the comparative strengths and weaknesses they display in certain processes assumed to underlie language functioning – e.g. auditory memory, sequencing and discrimination. Such taxonomies are instanced in many textbooks on language pathology, and the specific abilities approach is implicit in the theoretical model for the Illinois Test of Psycholinguistic Abilities (Kirk, McCarthy and Kirk, 1968). The categorical model also tries to typify the language characteristics of the various aetiological groups, and so might talk of the language of the deaf (Charrow, 1974 and Nickerson, 1975), of Down's syndrome children (Fraser, 1978) or the emotionally disturbed (Shapiro, Chiarandini and Fish, 1974). In as far as diagnostic labels do not tell a clinician or teacher how a child is developing language and therefore what intervention strategies need to be applied, their linguistic relevance is limited. If correctly handled they can give important indications as to why a child's linguistic profile has taken a particular form, and how remediation will need to be administered by taking into consideration other aspects of the syndrome (limits of amplification, mental age, hyperactivity, motivation, etc.). The influence of the medical model has been in the past not unresponsible for the attitude to bilinguals' behaviour as being somehow a 'disease' that needs to be overcome. Notwithstanding the (potential) bilingual is not immune from the causes of partial-hearing, cerebral palsy, specific learning disabilities and the like, and so are to be expected among the population of these categorically determined groups.

The medical model concentrates on signs and symptoms as pointers to underlying pathology in disorders and as such offers valuable information on the overall history of a child and his language problems. However, while such an approach may lend itself to the effective treatment of the causes of bacterial infections and prolapsed intervertebral discs, the causes of language disorders, even if discernible, are seldom amenable to direct treatment. There are as yet no tablets for *wh*-question development, nor injections to selectively suppress fronting in phonology. The analogy might not ring so ridiculous when one remembers many of the well-intentioned compensatory education programmes which sought to remedy Black English and Inner-city English by dealing children extra large doses of standard language input. For these reasons, in latter years, facilitated by advances in descriptive linguistics and child language studies, language clinicians and educationalists have come to favour the linguistic (Bloom and Lahey, 1978, Ch. 11) or behavioural (Crystal, 1980, p. 17) philosophy of analysis.

This method takes as its starting point the child's current language status, irrespective of how it arrived there, analyses the structures and processes as part of a description of the child's system and plans intervention on the basis of this and its relationship to the target (adult) language. Assessment procedures by Crystal *et al.* (1976) and Lee (1974) utilising the linguistic orientations were mentioned above. The rationale behind this states that for deaf, mentally-retarded, neurologically-impaired and normal child alike, the aim remains the same – mastery of the adult language. The ultimate aetiology may affect how material is presented, but not what is presented, since the model is the same for all, and as Bloom *et al.* (1978, p. 524) remark, 'At present, there is no reason to suspect that the sequence in which the model is achieved does, or should, differ for different groups of children.' Similarly Morehead (1975, p. 47) has stated that 'We now have considerable evidence in both language and cognition that deficient children do not organise these (syntactic, semantic etc.) systems in ways that are fundamentally different from those used by normal children.' Dulay *et al.* (1978) suggest that the acquisition 'errors' of bilingual children are not fundamentally different from those of monolingual learners, either. Thus, to this extent, the same type of learner problems and deviations from the norm can be expected among bilingual children, and, with the necessary adjustments to accommodate their differing linguistic environment, remediation content (as opposed to application) should also be essentially the same.

In characterising disordered language the behavioural approach does not primarily seek to establish the features of deaf language or whatever, but rather to focus on the acquisition process, the strategies used by children, the ways in which these develop non-normally and the type of language this produces. There is a dearth of serious literature dealing directly with this topic in bilingual children, in comparison to that written on monolinguals' disorders – though this latter has arisen only over the last decade. Most of the extant bilingual literature relates to second-language acquisition in later childhood and/or more formal settings. Some of this is mentioned below.

Describing Non-normal Variation

The linguistic orientation offers a framework within which language problems can be analysed, both for bi- and monolinguals. Bloom and Lahey (1978) along with many others divide language functioning into form (the lingusitic system – grammar, lexicon and phonology), content (conception and ideas of objects and events in the world) and use (how, where, when the form and content are applied). Normal acquisition results from proper development within these fields and, importantly, the correct interaction between the three. An individual's language in this way can be described according to the prime area of deficit and mis-interaction.

Following such a framework, a child might show acceptable levels of ideas about the world and events therein, and how to communicate them, but lack the adequate means to formulate these lexically or grammatically. Typically, in his play, such a child would demonstrate normal development of non-verbal patterns and general awareness, but would not have a formal system of expression to match this, having to rely heavily on gesture, and adapting what form he does command, to cover the shortfall. Normal children frequently experience periods where content development outstrips form (see for instance Grieve and Hoogenraad (1976) discussing chiefly lexical over-extension), and some language disorders may arise when such a gap, for whatever reason, develops. This behaviour is also typical of the bilingual child who has developed competence in one language, has a knowledge of how language is used and the world works, but does not sufficiently command his L2 (or L1 in some cases – see below) to convey his ideas and wishes. Attempts to communicate may come over as what is frequently labelled 'foreigner talk'.

There is great intersubject variation in how well individuals can make their limited language work for them, and it is erroneous always to equate the levels of development of form with ability to communicate, stressing the significance in assessment of not only seeing what the child *cannot* do, but also what he *can* do. It is those who do not succeed in reaching an effective level of linguistic improvisation that are likely to appear in the speech clinic or remedial language groups.

Of course saying that a child has a deficit in the field of form is not to assign a diagnostic label. To arrive at a symptomatic diagnosis it is necessary to specify the kinds of behaviour within the broader category that are bringing about deficient communication. This involves assessment of perceptual and analytical skills and processing and formulation strategies.

Within the field of form Crystal (1981, pp. 43-5), Grunwell (1982, pp. 184-92) and Ball (this volume) have discussed non-normal development of the phonological component. Crystal (1981, pp. 109-16, 185-91), Bloom *et al.* (1978, pp. 317-22) and Morehead (1975) give overviews of the study of deficient grammar in monolinguals while Dulay and Burt (1974a, b), Swain and Wesche (1975), McLaughlin (1977) and Kessler (this volume) are among those that deal with bilinguals. It should be noted that most bilingual studies are addressed to normal children, usually in formal school settings and as such still beg the question of differential diagnosis between second-language learning difficulty, where this occurs, and genuine language disorder. The general consensus is, however, that normal L2 acquisition resembles that of L1 with learning errors derived from common underlying learning strategies, while interference between the two languages constitutes only a small percentage of errors. This point is expanded later.

A different picture of disorder emerges when form and use are developing normally, but content lags behind. As the conceptual processes prerequisite for the development of content are also those that underlie the development of form and use, the presenting profile may be one of overall delay in passing linguistic milestones. Overall delay, however, seldom results in all subsystems of language development being equally retarded.

Another manifestation of content deficit is the so-called 'cocktail party' syndrome (Tew, 1979) where communication is typified by an intact phonological system, and appropriate conversational interaction, but the well-formed sentences contain a high percentage of stereotyped and overlearned phrases, with little informational load and a poverty of ideas. To the casual listener this can be deceptive, with a good accent and proper grammar giving superficially an impression of coping. A common manifestation of poor second-language control may also present as cocktail party-like conversation, where with phonological and syntactic fluency a child is able to rhyme off a limited set of social niceties or insults but little beyond this (compare the discussion in this and other chapters, of basic interpersonal communication skills v. cognitive/academic language proficiency).

Hymes (1971) called the knowledge needed for persons to handle the linguistic form and content at their command communicative competence. Acquiring the conventions of usage for a language are as much a part of development as the acquisition of the expresssion of negation or tense. There are children who have the formal means and underlying concepts to express themselves, but fail because they lack the necessary social skills or will.

In extreme cases, such as amongst elective mutes or autistic children, there may be no attempt made to communicate. With other affective syndromes, with institutionalisation or hyperactive children, usage might prove stereotyped, irrelevant to the topic at hand, or lacking in a coherent train of exchanges. Leudar (1981) and Prutting (1982) have discussed maladaptive aspects of usage. In as far as social interaction starts from the earliest months and it is on this development that later verbal development rests, the importance of the assessment and remediation of social exchange is reinforced. Early utterances rely heavily on non-verbal dimensions and so can be expected to be highly susceptible to impairment if use of these factors is outside of normal. Research in pragmatics and language disorders is embryonic, but one might speculate that it could become a very fruitful field in the search for what causes and maintains delayed onset of verbal language, deviant strategies and abnormal processes.

Language usage does not only cover gaze, turn-taking, initiating and terminating exchanges and appropriateness of form and content, it also involves exploiting the possible functions of it to enquire of, tell to and regulate others. One facet of usage that has long been recognised as a source of impairment to children is the failure they meet in situations where the pragmatics of communicating are outside their experience. The classical example is the switch from home to school with the attendant change in the functions of language and the expectations regarding what is accepted by teachers as the 'correct' usage for the pedagogical situation. These problems have been touched upon in the multicultural context by Perera (1981), Wiles (1981) and Twite (1981). In school, children have to learn different ways of meaning. Usage for reading and writing poses yet another new departure. Anderson (this volume) covers the full implications of this. Berdan (1981) discusses factors hindering the acquisition of literacy for Black English speakers related to usage, which are equally pertinent to the bilingual child.

Problems arising out of differences in the rules of communicative competence do not only pose difficulties in the switch from home to school. Any new situation that demands an alternative pragmatic set can lead to a breakdown in communication. This could include the language of the white test and tester, clinical consultations, or the instructions given for remediation. Differences also interfere in everyday interaction. Gumperz (1977) quotes two clear examples of misinterpretation of stress and intonation cues leading to misunderstanding and potential aggression between a West Indian busdriver and Asian canteen workers in London and their British English-speaking customers. Rules governing caste interaction may influence the type and amount of communication between children in a multi-ethnic classroom. Adler (1981) provides data on the contrasts in prosodic and paralinguistic features that can lead to misunderstandings and misdiagnoses in cross-cultural encounters.

Wide cultural variation exists in the regulation of speech, of entries, exits, interruptions and topic changes (Philips, 1976 and Kochman, 1981). Variation also exists in the uses to which language is put and its role in society. One particular aspect of this which could easily lead to misdiagnoses of language disorder is the use of silence. In Britain and North America, generally, to be verbally fluent, though not verbose, is socially prestigious, while to be silent, especially when introduced to someone for the first time, when a relationship/situation is ambiguous, or at parties, would be impolite and interpreted as rudeness, disinterest or distress. In the bilingual assessment context it may be misinterpreted as non-comprehension or as inability to respond. Testers would need to be assured that the subcultural acceptable silence was not masking a true language disorder.

Within the British-American cultural sphere, too, there are times when silence is appropriate, as for instance during solemn (religious) ceremonies, in libraries, and, as taught to many children, in the presence of adults, especially a stranger in what is seen as a socially higher ranking position. This might include clinicians and educationalists. A main source of dissatisfaction in medical consultations stems from the clinicians' reluctance to impart detailed explanations, but also from the consultees' reticence for social-interactive reasons to interrupt, request information, discuss matters they have not been asked about and question decisions made. Dumont (1972) examined the silence of Sioux and Cherokee children and the misinterpretation of this by white teachers, while Basso (1970) described the respect of silence amongst Western Apaches in family reunions, courtship and encounters between strangers. A contrast to this was reported by Reisman (1974) in Antigua, where conversational rules seemed anarchic compared even with the pressure to talk exerted by British-American conventions.

There were apparently no constraints on how many people would be talking simultaneously; pauses and eye contact were not signalled to permit another to join in or leave. One simply started speaking when one felt ready, and if there was no success at joining the exchange, one repeated the opening remark until heard by someone, or gave up.

There are many more aspects of use which it is not possible to cover in this limited context, such as the changes demanded by the switch from spoken to written usage, or later changes in school language style accompanying the move from primary to secondary education, or in the contrast between a history and a physics lesson. As well as deficient functioning in one of the main areas of the form-content-use triad, it is conceivable, exploiting that model further, that two other forms of disordered language would be theoretically feasible. The first would be a disordered interaction of the three categories in the presence of apparent normality of each.

J, a six-year-old boy, seen by the author, in a picture-naming exercise of familiar street objects, gave replies such as 'Is J going to post a letter' for a letterbox and 'I think he'll catch that man who robbed the bank' for a policeman. In that he was cooperating well in the task and held long conversations (all in language similar to the examples) with people he could give the impression of communicating well; the form of his utterances was well developed; and taken in isolation sensible content was expressed. However, while his overall intentions are clear none of the components matches appropriately to the form, content or usage required of the situation.

The opposite of this would be complete dissociation of the three components. Bloom *et al.* (1978) characterise these cases as portraying utterances that have minimal or no connection with the contexts in which they occur, are spoken at inappropriate times and use structures which have only chance relevance to any seemingly intended communication.

Problems with Bilingualism

Much emphasis has been given to the acquisition of the L2, but less attention has been devoted to the fate of L1 after L2 onset and the importance of L1-L2 interaction in the ongoing well development of both. Under optimum conditions children gain fluency in two, three or even four languages. Needless to say not all conditions provide the best climate, the latter being seldom for purely linguistic reasons, and more likely for social or psychological ones. It is in the less than ideal atmosphere that problems are produced – produced in the sense that from an isolated linguistic point of view there may be nothing untoward, but the variety of interaction between, and independent development of the two languages, set in the wider cultural context, may present a 'problem' with regard to the language expectations and demands placed on the individual.

In certain circumstances there are varying amounts of disruption to L1 learning after L2 onset which ranges from a delaying of development, through interrupted development, to complete dissolution of the L1. This in turn has repercussions for the L2. Aspects of bilingual acquisition have been covered in Chapters 2 and 3, but are mentioned here in the context of decisions on language intervention.

If L1 development is merely slowed – be it for reasons associated with the added cognitive load imposed by L2 onset, or as a result of the diminished functional importance of L1 and attention paid to it, the picture is one of continuing L1 acquisition but at a lesser rate. Thus, although progress in the child, if measured against monolingual norms, may be seen to be falling further and further behind, where there exists strong support for maintenance of L1 in the family or community, this comparative delay is unlikely to be significant, and the child's language system overall (L1 plus L2) is likely to form a communicative whole. The two languages in such circumstances develop along a functionally differentiated pattern, though there is usually some overlap.

According, however, to the degree of continued L1 support, its fate may be less than favourable. Progress may become so delayed that acquisition proceeds in an uneven manner. New items will probably be added to the lexicon, but the more complex syntactic and morphophonemic processes are never mastered and in effect the child's L1 development arrests at the age of L2 onset. A more extreme, but not unusual, occurrence associated with situations of active and benign discrimination against the L1, where few or no factors operate to maintain the language, is that L1 acquisition not only arrests, but with time gradually regresses in development as L2 use takes over. This dissolution may take place over months or years. In such cases expressive language suffers first, with the child maybe keeping a passive command a lot longer. The necessity, in assessing the child's communicative competence, of studying the family's attitudes to L1 maintenance and development and the nature of the child's L1 usage and knowledge is hereby stressed.

A further complication arising with the loss of L1 at a stage when L2 is only basically acquired, is that the child is severely disadvantaged alongside L2 monolinguals who have had several years' experience in the language. This disadvantage is liable to be more emphasised, in that L1 loss tends to go hand in hand with settings where there is no provision for L1 support in the schools and community. With extra English as a second language assistance the normal child may catch up with its monolingual counterparts. However, the danger exists of the L2 knowledge always lagging behind the level of conceptual expression and verbal insight required for success in the school curriculum.

Cummins (1980) has drawn a distinction between language proficiency at the level of basic interpersonal skills, which is achieved by everyone except severely subnormal and autistic people, and cognitive academic language proficiency (CALP) which is required for verbal reasoning, reading and other 'linguistic manipulation' tasks. He estimates that it requires at least five to seven years' length of residence in a country or experience with its language after the age of six before an adequate level of CALP is gained.

The language proficiency of children who have arrested or regressing L1 acquisition and L2 development that never manages to fulfil the demands placed on it have been labelled semilinguals (Skutnabb-Kangas and Toukomaa, 1976, 1980; Cummins, 1979; Brent-Palmer, 1979). The factors that bring about, and are associated with, semilingualism have strong implications for the relationship between bilingualism, cognitive development and academic achievement. These have been reviewed by Ben-Zeev (this volume), Swain and Cummins (1979) and in the works just cited and will not be repeated at this juncture. However, two further related notions, advanced, amongst others, by Cummins (1979) are relevant to assessment and intervention with the bilingual. These are the threshold and developmental interdependence hypotheses.

The threshold hypothesis claims that for there to be no negative effects on cognitive growth associated with delayed (bilingual) language development, a certain level of language proficiency must be attained. This is not an absolute level, but changes with the varying demands made on a child's linguistic systems through life. To benefit from the reported advantages of being bilingual an even higher threshold has to be reached. If the lower threshold is not reached the result is semilingualism.

The developmental interdependence hypothesis views L2 acquisition as being influenced by the level of L1 competence pertaining at the time of initial intensive L2 exposure. Effective L2 learning is considered to be facilitated by a high level of formal and conceptual development in L1. In contrast, where L1 skills are less well- or underdeveloped, intensive L2 exposure is seen as an impediment to further L1 development, which in turn sets a limit on the speed and extent of the L2 acquisition. It is in this light that poor school achievement of minority group children must be studied. From the same observations the strong arguments in favour of mother-tongue teaching have been derived (see Tosi, 1979c, and this volume; Saifullah-Khan, 1980).

Semilingualism can arise in normally developing children. For the language-disordered child the danger of falling into this state is all the more probable. The child who has a substantial delay in L1 acquisition resulting from an underlying disorder (in addition to or as opposed to sociocultural determinants in low-grade language exposure) is not likely to succeed in his L2. One must consider in fact whether or not these cases constitute a bilingual problem or should be treated as an L1 disorder. The issue also has implications for the language of remediation, a point that will be taken up in Chapter 10.

It has been pointed out that code-switching or mixing, when this occurs in the community as a whole, does not constitute a bilingual problem. It may be a problem for the monolingual listener, analyst or therapist, but that is another matter. There are, though, children who do not acquire the degree of metalinguistic awareness prerequisite for separating out the respective languages and where code-mixing does constitute a problem.

The ways in which languages are mixed are not random, but follow strict rules (Pfaff 1979). Different communities also maintain (consciously or unconsciously) levels beyond which, for any one situation, mixing is considered unacceptable. As yet no norms exist for any communities in relation to the types or levels of mixing, but it is research in this area that will be useful when making judgements on the normality of code differentiation. When developmental sequences in code differentiation and the types of mixing that are developmentally normal are identified we will stand in a better position to assess and remedy cases where abnormal mixing exists. McLaughlin (1977), Lindholm and Padilla (1978), Volterra and Taeschner (1978), Garcia (1980) and Harrison and Piette (1980) have written on areas close to this.

Examples of mixing have been interpreted by some as the influence of L1 on L2 (or vice versa) and errors have been understood as interference arising out of operating with two languages. Considerable controversy has reigned over how far this is true and how far 'errors' have sources other than interference. The controversy has implications for remediation in so far as it points either in the direction of specific language drills or developmental strategy teaching.

Error as Interference?

Along with the upsurge in interest in second-language teaching during the 1940s and 1950s there emerged under the influence of experience in this field and the influence of the then predominating behaviourist psychological accounts of language-learning, a view of second-language acquisition and teaching which laid great emphasis on the contrasts, in phonological, morphological and syntactic structure, between the native language of a speaker and any other language to be learned.

Generally behaviourist principles stated that language-learning, along with all other types of learning, was a matter of habit formation, the laying down of stimulus-response patterns from one's experience of external events. These principles further stated that if at any stage an organism was to learn a new response to a particular stimulus or a stimulus-response pattern closely related to a previously learned association, then the first response would require extinction before being replaced by the new response. During the period of learning or re-learning it was contended that prior habits would either facilitate subsequent learning, if the tasks were similar, or interfere with learning should there be differences, or, as it was frequently expressed, there would be a negative transfer. In other words, despite the new stimulus, the response would for a time, until complete reconditioning had taken place, maintain elements of the old habit or response.

Transferred to second-language learning, this mode of hypothesising predicted that the habits of the first language, i.e. the articulatory settings and perception of acoustic features of the other language, the syntactic patterns, morphological structure and semantic aspects of usage, would negatively influence a person's endeavours to produce or understand utterances in a second language, in as far as there might be differences between the languages in any of these systems or subsystems. Theoretically, where the two languages employed identical or similar structures – e.g. word order or tense marking – there would be ease of learning, while the greater the variations faced the more likely difficulties were to be expected.

Empirical evidence appeared to support this contention. 'Foreign' accent was interpreted in terms of failure to extinguish former phonological habits. Workers pointed to examples such as German learners of English declaring '*I live here since three years*' parallel to *Ich wohne seit drei Jahren hier* as evidence of negative transfer. Two works published in the early 1950s appeared to offer further confirmation. Weinreich (1953) systematically analysed the utterances of bilinguals and bidialectals and showed how seeming anomalies in their production of L2 could be described in terms of transfer of rules, or as he labelled it, interference from L1. Haugen's (1953) investigations of Norwegian in America brought to light similar findings.

The logical sequence to all this seemed to be that if *errors*, as they were then considered, in learning a second language were likely to occur at those points where the structures or processes of the native and target language differed, then by a systematic comparing, or contrasting, of the systems and subsystems of any two languages to highlight variations, learner difficulties or errors could be predicted. Further, teaching programmes could be designed that concentrated their drills on the expected problem areas. Thus, for instance, Fries, in his *Teaching and Learning English as a Foreign Language*, University of Michigan Press, Ann Arbor, 1945 (p. 9) whose work exerted much influence on the development of second-language teaching, wrote 'The most effective materials are those that are based upon a scientific description of the language to be learned, carefully compared with a parallel description of the native language of the learner.' Similarly Fries, in his foreword to another highly influential work in the field, Lado (1957), declared 'Learning a second language . . . constitutes a very different task from learning the first language. The basic problems arise not out of any essential difficulty in the features of the new language themselves but primarily out of the special "set" created by the first language habits', or as he had previously termed them 'blind spots' that prevent him (the learner) from responding to features that do not constitute the contrastive signals of his native language.

Lado (1957) stated in his preface that the plan of his work rested 'on the assumption that we can predict and describe the patterns that will cause difficulty in learning, and those that will not . . . by comparing systematically the language and culture to be learned with the native language and culture of the student', and that the significance of this for teaching was that (Lado, 1957, p. 2) 'the student who comes into contact with a foreign language will find some features of it quite easy and others extremely difficult. Those elements that are similar to his native language will be simple . . . those that are different will be difficult.'

All this served as a basis for the discipline of Contrastive Linguistics which dominated second-language teaching and learning and works on language 'problems' of bilingual children. However, the stance and claims of the 'Contrastive' field, and hence the nature of the relevance to the topic of language problems of bilingual children, has changed from the optimism of earlier decades *vis-à-vis* the prediction and solution of second-language difficulties. The notion that through Contrastive Analysis (CA) one can predict all difficulties a speaker of language A will encounter in acquiring language B, and set some scale of difficulty of structure according to by how many features the corresponding systems or subsystems in the two languages differ, has been labelled the strong version of the contrastive analysis hypothesis (Wardhaugh, 1970), while the modified version of the scope of the hypothesis, which, with debate still ongoing, most workers in the field would now confine themselves to, has come to be known as the weak version. The weak version rather than claiming predictive powers restricts itself to maintaining that certain aspects of L2 learners' usage can be accounted for by reference back to L1. Further it admits that not all 'errors' are necessarily a result of interference between L1 and L2 systems. Just what percentage of errors it might account for is disputed. James (1980, p. 146), in reviewing the literature on this, quotes between 36 and 51 per cent, though others (Dulay and Burt, 1974a) claim only 4.7 per cent.

The discrepancies in these percentages reflect in part difficulties that have arisen in upholding strong forms of the CA hypothesis and the subsequent rethinking that has been necessary. Another aspect concerns the level of interlanguage influence within the different levels of analysis. Some see interference as taking place mainly at the phonological level, while syntactic and semantic interference is much less. Depending on what data one uses, different readings will result.

Another dimension covers the distinction between what have been termed (Corder, 1971) covert and overt errors. Overt errors are those that are clear to the monolingual speaker, such as an Irish person stating *Is daddy in (the) garden* (on the basis of *tá daidí sa ghairdín*) when a statement *daddy is* is clearly intended. Covert errors are where statements appear normal on the surface but where the forms do not convey what the speaker intended, e.g. an English-speaker saying in German *Du musst nicht morgen kommen*, which is well formed, but an error if he intended to mean *You must not come tomorrow* rather than the less imperative *do not have to come* implication of *musst*.

Proponents of the CA hypothesis, even if they accept mixing as a normal part of bilinguals' language usage and second-language learning and not evidence of the negative effect of L1 on L2 have pointed to another body of data to support their contentions. This is the field of foreign language teaching and learning, where they have remarked that apparently typical errors can be isolated for Spanish or Hindi or Japanese learners of English that seem to be consistent across individuals and time – Jones (1979) and Jackson (1981).

Such claims have been criticised on two main fronts. The first is that far from easing the learning process for second languages, by locating areas of difference and supposed difficulty, many L2 learner errors may in fact be induced by the teaching strategy itself. This also brings into question the whole idea of grades of difficulty between particular languages as wholes, or certain subsystems within them.

One frequently hears the comment 'language x is a difficult language to learn, y is much easier'. Many lay English-speakers would claim that Samoan and Eskimo must present much greater problems in learning than, for example, Italian or Dutch. However, there is no evidence to confirm that Tibetan- or Lardil-speaking children or speakers of any of the so-called exotic languages take longer in acquiring their mother tongue than Portugese or English children. Neither is there any data showing differences in rate of acquisition, attributable to any inherent language or interlanguage difficulty of e.g. Chinese between English-Chinese bilinguals and Malay-Chinese bilingual children. There are differences reported regarding the age at which children of various languages acquire the adult form for expressing certain concepts (cf. de Villiers and de Villiers, 1979, p. 130ff) but these variations relate to intralanguage linguistic complexity for specific structures or subsystems. They do not relate to interlanguage overall differences. Similarly the apparent consistency of order of difficulty for learning certain English grammatical features for learners from several L1 backgrounds, and for L1 English children too (Day *et al.* 1978; Dulay and Burt, 1978) relates to English intralanguage linguistic complexity. Indeed, if any errors produced were derived from the respective L1s, one would have expected considerable variance. Hence 'exotic' is a subjective, relative label whose meaning is shaped by cultural, historical and social-affective factors rather than objective linguistic criteria.

Attempts to quantify distances between languages by reference to the degree of non-isomorphism measured in terms of the number of features (syntactic, phonological, etc.) by which they differ foundered on both theoretical, methodological grounds (what is to be measured against what and which models of description to use) and, as will be seen below, empirical grounds. The notion of exoticness and the prediction of difficulty in CA terms goes back to the pronouncements of Lado and Fries and (see above) is based on the idea that the less in common two languages have in the way in which something is expressed, the greater will be the task of learning between these two languages. Empirical evidence has not borne this out, and there appears to be no consistent correlation between assumed distance between languages and the degree of learning difficulty. In fact, Whitman and Jackson (1972), discussing the English errors of Japanese learners, concluded that 'relative similarity, rather than difference, is directly related to levels of difficulty'. Certainly from an impressionistic point of view in formal teaching contexts, minimal variation presents as much if not more of a problem than complete dissimilarity. This is a phenomenon not restricted to language-learning.

The second front on which second-language learning studies as support for the CA hypothesis has been criticised stems from highlighting differences between child and adult L2 learning. The majority of data used to uphold CA contentions were collected from formal classroom teaching situations with adolescent and adult students, not from children learning in natural settings or via the less formal teaching strategies of the early school years. Further, in interpreting the data, there was no real control of variables such as whether the subjects had previous (adult or childhood) L2 learning experience, whether they were students enrolled in college foreign language courses as opposed to, for instance, immigrants in reception classes or people attending adult education groups as a pastime. For such data to remain valid the hypothesis has to be upheld that adult L2 learning strategies are the same as child language-learning processes, and that the formal classroom contexts create the same learning environment as more naturalistic settings. Research has not confirmed this.

If the errors do not come from L1-L2 interference, there remains the question of where errors do arise. Implicit in the statements of Fries and Lado and their followers was an assumption that an L2 is learned through the filter of, and with constant reference to, the L1. An alternative hypothesis is that L1 and L2 learning share in common the underlying properties of the central nervous system and human cognitive functioning that enable humans to acquire language. Learning an L2 for pre-adolescents, in this view, takes place employing the same strategies that underlay L1 and hence any 'errors' will reflect not interference from the L1 but aspects of functioning or dysfunctioning of these underlying processes. Such a view has been strongly supported by Dulay and Burt (1974, a, b) and Dulay and Burt (1978).

These researchers analysed the productions of children acquiring an L2 and compared them with the types of error or goofs as Dulay and Burt (1974, a, b) have termed them produced by L1 learners. Their findings revealed that in the development of L2, utterances displayed few, if any, forms that could be unequivocally attributed to L1 influence. Rather productions were seen as displaying the same kind of gradual approximation to the adult language that can be seen in L1 development, and errors were more realistically interpretable in terms of the 'active mental organisation' and reorganisation of the language system that was taking place as the child constructed and tested out new hypotheses according to its stage of general cognitive development and language data available.

There have been several typologies advanced labelling the child's developmental productions, which despite using varying terminology, identify essentially the same phenomena. The similarity of these classes to those discussed above (p. 84) is not coincidental if one accepts the common underlying processes hypothesis. Dulay and Burt (1978) categorise the intralingually determined creative errors into six groups, namely overregularisation, omissions, use of archiforms, alternating use of the members of a class, double markings and misorderings.

J. Richards (1971) includes overgeneralisation, ignorance of rule restrictions, incomplete application of rules and false concepts hypothesised. This last category – also called induced errors (Stenson, 1975) and transfer of training by Selinker (1972) – refers to errors arising from teaching methods that concentrate on discrete supposed accident blackspots at the expense of an overall view of how structures or processes interact within a language as a whole. Learners through this concentration can be drawn on to rocks that they might not have struck had they not been lured on to them.

Conclusion

This chapter opened by stating that the notion 'problem' is a highly subjective area. It is subjective not because people who have a genuine language disorder do not exist, but because in the field of bilingualism, especially, there is to be found a range of variety in language greater than encountered elsewhere. There has been a tendency to label different as disordered. This is not confined to language studies, it being prevalent in mental health, social work and education, too. The aim here has been to highlight some of the types and causes of variety that in the past have been designated problems, in the hope that one is thereby better able to isolate genuine disorders and better able to plan intervention how, when and where necessary.

In striving for a more accurate view of language problems, several points of consideration were stressed. The first is an awareness of normal acquisition patterns, both the universal tendencies and the individual learning processes. Acquisition and use must be measured in relation to the child's own linguistic environment and how it functions, not according to how the clinician thinks it operates or ought to operate, nor in relation to the clinician's own linguistic norms. The purpose of assessment and remediation must be borne in mind – whether it is to gauge the stage of language development, to determine reasons for school failure, placement in a particular type of school, or whatever. All these will have a bearing on the weighting given to the various linguistic and extralinguistic factors, since the existence of prejudices and the effect they have on our everyday lives, however 'wrong' they may be, is a reality, and one cannot, as Hymes (1974a, p. 64) warns, 'blink realities' and inequalities simply because we have some ideological objection to them.

If we can be aware of our own prejudices we should be better able to judge which language difficulties are centred on the child's own development, and which ones are products of having to communicate in a society biased against him. It was mentioned above how attitudes to languages influence views of how and where they should be used and taught, and that many problems are created by misguided political-educational decisions, however well intentioned. Coard (1971), and Haberland and Skutnabb-Kangas (1979) have all drawn attention to different aspects of this.

The linguistic description and principled planning of language intervention with children identified as having a genuine language disorder has only begun to flourish over the past decade in the wake of advances made in the study of first-language acquisition. Studies in bilingual acquisition and usage are now sufficiently developing to enable an equal expansion of disordered acquisition studies in bilinguals.

Part 2

LANGUAGE ASSESSMENT

5 SOME OBSERVATIONS CONCERNING FORMAL TESTS IN CROSS-CULTURAL SETTINGS

Niklas Miller

The issues involved in cross-cultural assessment have been a strong focus in the controversies concerning racial and individual equality and inequality. Proponents in the age-old debate between the nature and nurturists have found confirmation of their views in the outcome of testing. Genetic determinists have taken the assignment of an inordinately high proportion of ethnic minority children to schools for the educationally subnormal (see Chinn, 1980, p. 50 and HMSO, 1981, p. 45) as evidence for innate racial inferiority, while environmental interactionists have linked these circumstances with the socio-economic and wider discrimination against such groups. Aside from the broader societal aspects of the debate, much argument has centred around the role of the Western notion of 'intelligence' and of the devising, administration and interpretation of assessment materials based on this notion, in supporting or distorting various views. It has been questioned whether or not 'intelligence' as a meaningful pure entity exists, and even if it does, whether it is accessible to quantification. If it is, then do the tests which purport to measure it succeed, and if not, what is it they are actually assessing? Is intelligence, as it has been cynically expressed, merely what intelligence tests measure, is it an artificial construct of value judgements related to what is considered necessary to succeed in Western society, is it so, as Anastasi and Foley (1949, quoted in Vernon, 1969, p. 89) have suggested, that 'The "higher" mental processes of one culture may be the relatively worthless "stunts" of another'? Or is there substance to the claims of workers like Eysenck (1973) and Jensen (1972) that what they define as intelligence is instrumental in creating the perceived interracial and individual differences?

Bias in Testing

The scientific and political polemics surrounding this issue have been amply covered elsewhere. Samuda (1975) is a general work dealing with multicultural assessment; Herman (1979) reviews research on the use of standardised tests to identify bilingual handicapped children;

Cleary *et al.* (1975), G. Jackson (1975) and Bernal (1975) represent opposing views on test usage with disadvantaged students. Ryan (1972) has examined the illusion of objectivity in attainment testing, while Daniels and Houghton (1972) and Henderson (1976) have drawn attention to the class function of testing and labelling. Space precludes here a full analysis of these arguments and their relevance for test validity, reliability, standardisation and interpretation. Further discussion is limited to highlighting some of the more obvious pitfalls in multicultural assessment.

Intellectual abilities do not develop independently of a person's environment, even if the initial underlying determinants of growth are theoretically isolatable within an individual. Neither, contrary to the pretence of the extreme proponents of the objectivity of IQ testing, does assessment take place in a vacuum, with candidates divesting themselves of all their cultural characteristics as soon as they sit down to a test. This point became only slowly acknowledged in the psychometric literature, and even more slowly in psychometric practice. Many factors intrinsic to the individual and test situation exercising a biasing influence were only gradually recognised.

The unfair advantages that seemed to help white middle-class Anglo-American and South-East English oriented children to favourable test results were seen to derive from the operational definitions of ability that were employed being directly related to the moral and intellectual values and expectations of these groups. Thus in the same way that Anglo children experienced a cultural continuity in the move from home to school, so also they were assessed in areas of performance in which they had been consciously and unconsciously brought up. Further, they were judged according to methods and yardsticks with which they were familiar. Testees from other cultural traditions who achieved poorly on these measures were labelled deficient, and later disadvantaged, but only recently in some quarters, with the rise of pluralist tolerance, have they been considered legitimately different and possessive of capabilities in their own right.

The cultural determinants of bias external to the tests themselves include general aspects of the environment, child-rearing and schooling differences and the sociocultural position and role of the test population within the society as a whole. Much has been made of the contrasts in attitudes to test-taking and response styles. In particular (e.g. Samuda, 1975, p. 85) tests and test ethos in stressing the individualistic, competitive, try your hardest, answer at all costs, 'hard-work' as being a means to a future end, and way of gaining the better of one's contemporaries which are cherished qualities of white middle-class upbringing are seen to discriminate against those communities tending to opposite values. Other communities might frown upon individualism as disrespect for the wisdom of elders or the collective decision-making role of the family or community group. Similarly striving to emulate one's peers in competition might be taken as betraying the communal spirit of mutual support and achievement of goals through common effort.

The expression of the puritan ethic of reaping eventual rewards (material, intellectual) through hard work contrasts sharply with cultures where the emphasis lies in applying oneself to fulfil more immediate demands. Therein lies also a contrast between those who can feel confident that through success in tests and other tasks they can win control of their destiny and environment and those who, even if they wished, are doubtful whether such individual application will produce benefits. The role of self-concept and its effect on motivation and achievement are widely documented (Stone, 1981). Apart from the possible unfamiliarity of non-Anglo-oriented children with test and test-like situations and their functions, those who have experienced failure or non-acceptance at the hands of majority culture education come to assessment situations not with the feeling that it is an occasion to forward their individual interests, but that it is yet another place where their inferiority and remoteness from the mainstream are going to be confirmed. Conversely the atmosphere, attitudes and contents of assessment to majority culture children will have a relevance and familiarity which will help them towards an optimum performance.

The atmosphere of the test is taken to include not only the cognitive and affective background that the child brings to the situation and the differential effects this has, but also more specific aspects of the event. Samuda (1975, p. 91) has highlighted the significance of reactions to physical setting as a variable in test scores. Quite often testing takes place as part of a special visit to an unfamiliar clinic (or in a special room set aside in a school) with all its attendant anxieties. More likely than not the tester will be a stranger to the child and parents. These factors apply equally to the majority culture child, but with the minority child there are the added influences of possible racial and language/dialect differences, and difficulties in the use of an alien health or education system.

Score-depressing factors more closely associated with the assessment procedure itself include the already mentioned orientation of some subgroups away from sitting down in formal or semiformal situations and cooperating in giving answers on their own individual initiative to questions they may realise the other person already knows the answer to. Likewise poor adjustment to the artificiality of assessment sessions, the unaccustomed use of paper and pencil, the pressure of time, the culturally determined tendency to either give a minimum response or to elaborate at length on topics have also been noted as causing a negative effect on results.

Alongside considerations of extra-test variables there are numerous factors intrinsic to tests which discriminate against certain groups. The most obvious, apart from language, is the use of culture-bound toys, pictures and general knowledge. Smith and Lawley (1948) in their measurements in Gaelic and English with children from the Outer Hebrides used materials that included pictures of trains, scooters, lamp-posts and watering cans which in the pre-television age were hardly likely to be familiar objects to those islanders. Dolls, teasets and cars which are heavily represented among test objects are not universal toys. Neither are apparently cross-cultural valid measures such as formboards, block design and object construction free from bias. Ortar (1963) classed such procedures amongst the most culture-bound, and Berry (1966) detected racial differences between Scots, Eskimos and members of the Temne tribe from Sierra Leone using such material. W. Hudson (1967) demonstrated how perception of pictures cannot be assumed to be uniform across cultures.

The most prominent component placing certain groups at a disadvantage is language. This does not only mean the belatedly recognised preposterousness of subjecting children to assessment in a language that is not their mother-tongue, as the language-centred problems are more deeply rooted than simply a matter of choice between language A or B. A recurrent theme throughout this book is that groups not only speak different languages, in the textbook grammar sense, but that through their view of the world and their social and psychological preferences they have different ways of meaning, of verbally conceptualising feelings and events, and different patterns of usage. Added to this are the prejudices attached to particular varieties (Chapters 1 and 3) and cross-cultural differences in paralinguistic signals (Chapters 3 and 4). The notion of semilingualism (Chapters 3, 4, 11) and Cummins's (1980) distinction between fluency at the level of 'basic interpersonal communicative skills' and full 'cognitive/academic language proficiency' also have direct relevance to testing. Cummins (p. 103) claimed that for children who arrive in a new linguistic environment after the age of six, the acquisition of age-appropriate L2 cognitive/academic language proficiency, the type of proficiency required in most tests, can take up to seven years. Thus examiners are warned not to presume that just because a bilingual child can chat coherently about everyday matters in their L1 or L2, that they can be tested on a par with monolingual speakers of the same languages.

Tests then are biased linguistically not only superficially, in whether they use language A or B and in the words they use, but more deeply in the linguistic structures and assumptions that underlie test construction and interpretation (cf. Taylor, 1977). The report, cited by Samuda (1975, p. 92), of the Committee on Hostile Test Center Environment found that 'a significantly greater percentage of minority (7%) than white students mentioned the failure to understand the instructions'. Grill and Bartel (1977) in analysing the grammatic closure subtest of the Illinois Test of Psycholinguistic Ability (Kirk *et al.*, 1968) identified twenty-three of the thirty-three items as potentially discriminating against non-standard dialect speakers. Similar examples could easily be found from many other tests.

Elimination of Bias in Testing

In response to the awareness of the inadequacies of traditional tests, various reforms have been attempted. Some of the modifications are on an *ad hoc* basis. Samuda and Crawford (1980, p. 131 and 232) found that 82.4 per cent of school boards surveyed by them made adjustments when testing ethnic minority students, the most frequent being time extension, omission of items and substitution of words or phrases. Evard and Sabers (1979), Chinn (1980) and Mowder (1980) have described approaches that have been made to cross-cultural assessment, including the use of culture-free and culture-fair tests, the modification of existing tests, criterion-referenced measures, creation of regional norms and the development of pluralistic assessment techniques. Hegarty and Lucas (1978, p. 74) also mention regression, constant ratio and conditional probability models as methods of producing fair scoring and selection across groups.

Culture-free testing assumed that beneath the nurture-influenced surface behaviour of an individual one could locate 'intelligence' in natural form, and the shortcomings of previous procedures stemmed from their failure to penetrate the culture-bound overlay. However, endeavours to create such a test all came to nought (see Samuda, 1975, and Hegarty and Lucas, 1978) and the search shifted towards a less ambitious culture-fair goal.

Tests devised as culture-fair sought to remove procedures and items that were deemed discriminatory against certain groups, and concentrated on methods and measures that were presumed to be uniform across communities. Verbal sections were either fully dropped or de-emphasised and prominence was given to constructional and visual-spatial tasks with instructions issued orally or in mime. Alternatively or additionally scoring procedures were adapted to give equal weighting to various subgroups. These reforms met with little more success than the culture-free aims. Tests such as Raven's Progressive Matrices, and the Goodenough-Harris draw-a-man test, though an improvement on earlier measures, were shown nevertheless to contain cultural bias – see Samuda (1975, p. 138), and the discussion above regarding cultural differences in object manipulation and pictorial perception. The rigorous pruning of unfair aspects left psychometrists with severely limited instruments with respect to the breadth of information that could be gleaned on an individual's or group's ability and potential.

Further efforts to resolve the cross-cultural assessment dilemma centred on the translation of entire tests or the use of interpreters to permit administration or responses in different languages. This enabled a more accurate appraisal for some groups (see Swanson and De Blassie, 1979) but this strategy far from removes all cultural bias. Translating a test only alters the language; it does not change the culturally weighted nature of the theory of intelligence on which items were designed, nor the discriminatory non-verbal content, either of the materials, or the expected replies. Neither does it remove the negative self-concept that the child may bring to the test situation, nor the effects of wider environmental discrimination and the level of motivation associated with these. Howard (1982) points out the hidden bias in digit recall, even if one does permit the child to reply in his L1. An instance of differences in expected answers is given in Howard's example of the translation into Spanish of the WISC question 'What is the thing to do when you cut your finger?' His Costa Rican subjects, having recovered from the shock of the translation which insinuates the finger has been completely severed, typically responded with 'put coffee grounds on it', that being local practice. N. Miller (1978) mentions the problems associated with the translation of kinship and colour terminology and the cultural variation that exists in attitudes to the roles of different family members, or the differing importance of animals as pets, food and in utility. Translating items can alter the difficulty of questions. As Miller (1978) also stressed, a concept may be expressed in L1 by a linguistically simple structure, but the same concept (comparative, negation, etc.) in L2 requires a complex structure.

Another complicating factor ignored by the apparently easy solution of translating all or parts of tests is the nature of a bilingual's language usage. Testing a child in L1 assumes that his mastery of that language is comparable to monolingual L1 speakers. It also takes for granted that the forms of L1 and L2 the child uses are the standard varieties. This may be far from the case. It also assumes even development of all components in a given language. This also may be far from true. It is quite possible for a child to have age-appropriate command of L1 syntax but delayed lexical development in that language, while the position is reversed for his L2. A child's knowledge of L1 might be adequate for family and shopping affairs but be poor for discussing his emotions or for verbal reasoning. Gerken (1978) amongst others has established the importance of language dominance as a variable in test outcome.

The quest for a cirumvention of the culture trap has led to departures from reformist attempts to remove bias from tests. One direction has exploited the construction of tests specifically geared and standardised to the social and linguistic world of a given community, judging a child with his own cultural peers rather than white middle-class values. The System for Multicultural Pluralistic Assessment (Mercer and Lewis, 1978) represents an example of this 'pluralistic sociocultural' direction. This approach has considerable potential, although the heterogeneity of most subgroups renders problematical a complete fairness. It does not surmount the obstacle of wider discrimination against minorities in society either.

Another departure has been to leave behind the selection and prediction functions of traditional testing in favour of descriptive and prescriptive models. This move marks a change from viewing subjects on norm-scales, in comparison to whatever population, and deriving predictions about future performance on the basis of past learning as instanced by a candidate's performance on a test. In its stead, the diagnostic-prescriptive model (e.g. Chinn, 1980, p. 59) treats each child as an individual with a learning potential. Rather than evaluate this potential from a static IQ score, an effort is made to measure the dynamic processes by which the child learns, the rate at which he learns and those areas in which he learns better or worse. Hegarty and Lucas (1978) have examined learning ability as a means for diagnosis and the planning of intervention.

Conclusion

The foregoing has been only an all too narrow overview of some of the issues involved in the debate on multi- and cross-cultural assessment. For more detailed debate readers are referred to the works mentioned and the extensive writing on testing in the psychological literature. If one were to draw any conclusion from the above points, it would be that intelligence as conceived in Western culture cannot be viewed independently of the sociocultural constructs which contribute to its shaping, nor independently of the cultural content of the verbal and non-verbal means available to 'measure' it. Agreeing with Hegarty and Lucas (1978, p. 35), 'In the absence of a comprehensive account of how measured intelligence is related to sociocultural and ethnic difference, IQ scores have to be regarded in a very tentative light . . .' A way forward out of the testing impasse would seem to be offered in a return to descriptive models, which prescribe placement and judgements on the basis of what a child can and cannot do from an analysis of his own systematic behavioural function.

Such a stance does not imply the complete rejection of formal attainment tests. Properly used, they can supply a large amount of specific information in a short space of time, they can be effectively employed in monitoring change and establishing a child's ability relative to his peers. What is advised against is not their use, but their abuse in construction, execution and interpretation. When prudently applied in conjunction with other independent measures they can act as a valuable tool in the assessment, placement and teaching processes.

6 PHONOLOGICAL DEVELOPMENT AND ASSESSMENT

Martin Ball

The acquisition of phonology has received much attention within the field of developmental linguistics, and much data has been collected. This has usually been in the form of individual 'diary studies' or 'case studies' (see for example Francis, 1975, for reports on these; for a more modern case study see N. Smith, 1973). However, researchers have not agreed on how to characterise the development of phonology theoretically. In earlier studies (see for example McLaughlin, 1978, for reports on these in the bilingual situation), phonological development was viewed from the standpoint of classical phonemics (see Jones, 1951), and the acquisition of the sound system of a language considered to be accomplished in much the same way as the analysis of the system into phonemes. That is, that the child acquires individual phones which eventually become grouped into contrastive units (i.e. phonemes), and that more and more phonemes are acquired, until eventually the phonemic system of the adult language is achieved. For details on a chronology of phoneme development in English see Grunwell (1982). Most evidence seems to suggest that in terms of phoneme acquisition, nasals and plosives appear first; bilabial and alveolar are the first place distinctions, followed by velar. Fricatives, affricates and liquids appear later, with interdental fricatives being among the last phonemes to appear (see Figure 6.1).

However, as Grunwell (1982) points out, such an approach tells us nothing about phonological structure, that is to say about where in syllable structure the phonemes first appear (in fact it tends to be in initial position), and about the development of phoneme combinations. Such information obviously also needs to be provided. Another criticism levelled at the phoneme-by-phoneme approach is that it is uneconomical and non-insightful. Therefore, although we can say that on average between the ages of 1;6 and 2;0 a child acquires the phonemes /m, p, b, n, t, d/, we are missing an insight into the relationship between the sounds. If we concentrate instead on describing those features that are common between the sounds and those that serve to distinguish them, we can say that the child has acquired the following phonetic features which he is using phonologically (i.e. contrastively): nasality, plosivity, voicing, bilabial place, alveolar place. Various schemes of

Figure 6.1: Phoneme Acquisition

	0;9 – 1;6	1;6 – 2;0	2;0 – 2;6	2;6 – 3;6	3;6 – 4;6	4;6 +
NASAL	nasal	m n	m n (ŋ)	m n ŋ	m n ŋ	m n ŋ
PLOSIVE	plosive	pb td	pb td (kg)	pb td kg	pb td kg tʃ dʒ	pb td kg tʃ dʒ
FRICATIVE	(fricative)		h	f s h	fv sz ʃ h	fv θð sz ʃʒ h
APPROXIMANT	(approximant)	w	w	w j (l)	w j l (r)	w j l r

phonological distinctive features have been drawn up (see Hyman, 1975, or Sommerstein, 1977), the first by Jakobson, Fant and Halle (1952); and Jakobson himself, amongst others, has used the system to describe phonological acquisition (Jakobson, 1942; see also Winitz, 1969).

Developed after distinctive feature theory (and in some respects incorporating it), generative phonology as proposed by Chomsky and Halle (1968), has also been used to characterise phonological development, e.g. by N. Smith (1973). It is not necessary for our purposes to go into this topic deeply (see Grunwell, 1982), and we need only note that the theory can be used to state a series of *phonological rules* relating various stages of development to the adult model, the rules being deleted or adapted or added to at the different stages.

The most recent, and perhaps the most insightful, way of characterising phonological development is that termed *natural phonology* or *phonological process theory*. This has built on insights provided by the previously mentioned approaches, but also has long roots. As long ago as 1922, Jespersen noted that phonological acquisition went through a series of 'strictly observed sound-laws' (p. 107), but it was not until recently that these phonological processes have been described in depth (Ingram, 1976, 1979; Grunwell, 1982). As a method of characterising the development of phonology this method has several advantages: not only are generalisations captured by avoiding the phoneme-by-phoneme approach, but structural considerations enter into the analysis as well – for example, in the processes dealing with consonant clusters. The theory also has a stronger (and controversial) claim: that phonology is governed by a set of universal phonological processes which are innate (for further discussion of this point see Grunwell, 1982). Acquisition is seen as the use of certain phonological processes at certain stages of development, which are dropped or changed at a later stage. Figure 6.2 shows the development of natural phonological processes, though as with all such dating of phonological development the stages are norms, and there is much individual variation as well as idiosyncratic processes.

However, it is clear that phonological development will be different to some extent in a bilingual situation, because the phonological patterns of two or more languages are being acquired. Precisely how this affects phonological acquisitions depends on several factors. First, it is important to note the distinction between simultaneous acquisition of the two (or more) languages, and successive acquisition (L1 followed by L2). Baetens-Beardsmore (1982) points out that in terms of

Figure 6.2: The Development of Phonological Processes

0;9 – 1;6	1;6 – 2;0	2;0 – 2;6	2;6 – 3;0	3;0 – 3;6	3;6 – 4;6	4;6 +
All processes can apply, individual consonant variation,	reduplic., cons. harmony, final cons. deletion, cluster reduction.	final cons. deletion, cluster reduction.	final cons. deletion, cluster reduction.	clusters with liquids appear.	clusters become established	
phonetic variability	velar fronting; stopping; liquid gliding, context sensitive voicing	(velar fronting); stopping; liquid gliding, context sensitive voicing	stopping of /v ð z tʃ dʒ/: /θ/→[f] /ʃ/→[s] liquid gl. context sens. voic.	stopping of /v ð (z)/; /θ/→[f] ; fronting of /ʃ tʃ dʒ/; liquid gliding.	/θ/→[f] /ð/→[d] / [v] liquid gliding.	(/θ/→[f] /ð/→[d] / [v] liquid gliding.)

phonological interference between L1 and L2, often 'the child or early bilingual has no problems here' (p. 60);[1] whereas the late bilingual may 'interpret and reproduce sounds of L2 according to relatively atrophied patterns developed for L1' (p. 60). For a fuller discussion on these types of L2 acquisition see McLaughlin (1978). The kinds of problems encountered in phonological interference will be returned to later.

A second important factor having a bearing on possible L1-L2 interference concerns the statuses of the languages being acquired. If we look at the example of a child acquiring Welsh and English in a Welsh-speaking area, whether or not this is simultaneous acquisition, the likelihood of *phonological* interference is small as both the languages he is learning possess a similar prosodic system and similar vowel and consonant realisations, with just a few differences in system and structure. He is learning a *Welsh* accent of English, not RP or any other variety.

On the other hand, if a child is for example acquiring French and German while living in France, phonological interference is more likely between the two, and as French would probably be the dominant language (though other factors are also important here), it would be most likely to have the greater effect on the phonology of the German being learnt. Examples might include the omission in German of post-vocalic nasals and the simultaneous nasalisation of the vowel ([man] –> [mã]), the loss of pre-vocalic glottal stop ([ʔerst] –> [erst]), and the change of rhythm from stress-timed to syllable-timed, among many other possibilities. The terms *primary* and *secondary* systems can be used to capture this distinction, where the *primary* system refers to the phonological system of the bilingual's dominant language (L1), and the *secondary* system to the bilingual's less dominant language (L2). Baetens-Beardsmore (1982, Chapter 3) discusses how dominance can be measured in bilinguals.

Apart from the area of interference, does the acquisition of two languages imply that identical phonological processes are used for both? Bellin (1983) looked at this question in a description of some of the processes he found in children learning Welsh and English. Whereas in certain cases similar processes operated in both languages, an instance is given where this was not so. It is noted that one of the children studied developed a process at the age of 3;10 whereby /θ/ and /ð/ were replaced by [s] and [z] respectively, in Welsh. At the same time, when speaking English, /θ/ and /ð/ were replaced by [f] and [v]. Although reasons for this difference can be advanced in terms of the functional load of the sounds in question, it nevertheless exemplifies the fact that different processes and different timescales may be involved in the acquisition of the two phonological systems.

Phonological Disorders

Various ways of classifying speech sound disorders have been used, but first the distinction must be clearly made between phonetic and phonological disorders. A phonetic disorder is one which does not upset the system of contrastive phonological units, for example where the normal pronunciation of a phoneme is substituted by a sound outside the system of the language. Grunwell (1982) gives the example of English /s/ being substituted by [ɬ]; as English does not contain a phoneme /ɬ/, no confusions would result. However if /s/ is substituted by [t], confusions would result, as there is a phoneme /t/ (/təu/-/səu/, etc), therefore this is termed a phonological disorder.

Phonetic disorders are mostly outside the scope of this chapter, so further consideration will now be given to the analysis of phonological disorders, and in particular developmental phonological disorders. Of course, to a large extent, errors tend to be classified according to the particular model of development that is espoused, i.e. in terms of phoneme errors, feature errors, misapplication of a generative rule (for example), and so forth. However, a closer look at some of the more widely used terms will be taken.

In the analysis of errors from a phonemic viewpoint, a common classification was into:

1. Omission of a phoneme.
2. Substitution of one phoneme by another.
3. Distortion of a phoneme (i.e. use of an unusual allophone, or phone not found in the language).
4. Addition of a phoneme.

(See Grunwell, 1982, for discussion of the development of this schema.) This sort of analysis could present a score of degree of disorder by simply counting the number of errors present in a sample of the patient's speech obtained via one of the standardised tests (see below), with some of the error types counting as worse than others (e.g. type 1 is considered worse than type 2, which in turn is worse than type 3). However, this approach often obscures important generalisations, and as Grunwell (1982) notes, 'provides no indication whatsoever as to the nature of a person's speech disorder and no guidance as to possible intervention strategies' (p. 64). A whole pattern of phonological changes could be obscured through this classification, leading to inappropriate treatment procedures.

Many of the other approaches to phonology outlined above did little more than refine these four patterns, still working within a framework of error analysis. A new classification of phonological disorders emerged with natural phonology which, although it does not supply a scoring system, does avoid many of the pitfalls of traditional error analysis. As already described, natural phonology involves the analysis of data according to a set of natural phonological processes, and it is these processes which can be assigned to different categories. At a basic level, the processes seem to divide between *delay* and *deviancy*: that is, between processes which normally occur in phonological development but have been retained longer than usual, and processes which do not normally occur in phonological development. However, it is doubtful whether our knowledge of what normally occurs is sufficient to make this a rigid distinction.

A more refined classification of disordered phonologies from the natural phonology viewpoint is given by Grunwell (1982), who proposes three main categories:

1. Persisting normal processes.
2. Chronological mismatch.
3. Unusual and idiosyncratic processes.

An example of the first type would be retention of a process such as cluster reduction beyond the period when it would normally be dropped. Chronological mismatch implies a child's speech which retains some processes normally dropped early on, with other developments characteristic of a later stage. The third category includes deviant processes, and ones peculiar to a particular child, including favourite articulation, whereby one sound or group of sounds is used extremely often with no apparent phonetic explanation.

The following data provide specific examples of these categories:

Persisting normal processes
Rhodri 5;6 (1979)

1.	[ɬam]	fflam	/flam/	6. [fov]	stove	/stov/
2.	[ˈfɪdjai]	sgidiau	/ˈsgɪdjai/	7. [ɬiv]	sleeve	/sliv/
3.	[kɪft]	clust	/klɪst/	8. [vɛf]	dress	/drɛs/
4.	[ˈɛftɪg]	esgid	/ˈɛsgɪd/	9. [dok]	goat	/got/
5.	[ˈkɛdɪl]	tegell	/ˈtɛgɛɬ/	10. [taɪk]	kite	/kaɪt/

These data show the continued use of processes normally lost by this age: cluster reduction (in examples 1, 2, 3, 6, 7, 8), and metathesis (in 4, 5, 9, 10). These examples also show a process whereby /s/ is realised as [f] (2, 3, 4, 6, 8). Some of the cluster reductions also show feature synthesis (e.g. /f/ + /l/ –> [ɬ] in 'fflam', also in 7).

Chronological mismatch
Gareth 4;7 (1980)

1. [tid]	cig	/kig/	5. [blat]	black	/blak/
2. [ˈprəni]	prynu	/ˈprəni/	6. [trim]	cream	/krim/
3. [tlus]	tlws	/tlus/	7. [brɪn]	bring	/brɪŋ/
4. [dlan]	glân	/glan/	8. [pleɪ]	play	/pleɪ/

These data illustrate the use of an immature process (velar fronting, in 1, 4, 5, 6, 7) together with the use of clusters (a later feature, seen in 2, 3, 4, 5, 6, 7, 8).

Unusual/Idiosyncratic processes
Gwyneth 3;5 (1982)

1. [ˈhoˀɪ]	llygoden	/ɬəˈgodɛn/	4. [taˀ]	tap	/tap/
2. [ˈmoˀɪ]	modur	/modɪr/	5. [hɐp]	shop	/ʃɐp/
3. [ˈpɛhə]	pedwar	/pɛdwar/	6. [ˈpaˀɪ]	party	/ˈpati/

These data illustrate the use of a 'favourite' articulation in both Welsh and English: glottal replacement (the use of [h] in 1, 3, 5; and the use of [ˀ] in 2, 4, 6).

The use of a process-based classification results 'in a more generalised and economical description of the differences between the target and error pronunciations because processes are defined as operating on classes of sounds' (Grunwell, 1982, p. 192). Traditional error analysis with its concentration on individual sounds can not of course be as insightful. A process analysis also gives specific guidelines to therapy, and this topic is discussed further below.

Assessment Procedures

In terms of assessing a speaker's phonological competence, the most usual method has been through the use of so-called *articulation tests.*

This term is an unfortunate one, implying as it does a purely articulatory phonetic interest, when the tests are designed to investigate phonology also. Traditionally, the design of these tests has involved the use of pictures to elicit specific words, the words having been chosen to include the phonemes and phoneme sequences of the language. However, limitations of time restrict the number of phonemes it is possible to include, and most tests concentrate on the consonants, examining them in initial, medial and final position; and include representatives of the most usual consonant clusters. The tests usually envisage an error-analysis approach to the data obtained.

This sort of approach is open to criticism, and Grunwell (1982) points out some of the design-related shortcomings. For example, the term *medial* is misleading, as a word-medial consonant can be either syllable-final within the word, or syllable-initial within the word. Furthermore, the concentration on a relatively small number of words (40 to 50 in most tests), and the fact that most phoneme targets appear only once can lead to an erroneous analysis. Grunwell (1982) also notes that the articulation test approach is usually very much a phoneme-by-phoneme error analysis, thereby obscuring wider patterns and effects occurring within particular words, or across word boundaries (e.g. assimilation). She sums up her views with three criteria for an adequate data base, which should be:

1. fully representative of system and structure;
2. able to portray different stylistic ranges;
3. obtained from differing situations (i.e. not just a test situation) (see p. 61).

However, she does feel that the articulation test can be of use in 'obtaining relatively rapidly a sample for a screening assessment' (p. 69-70).

Applying these criteria to the acquiring of data for an assessment of bilingual phonology suggests the following points:

1. To be fully representative the data should include examples of all the segmental units (i.e. phonemes) of the systems of all the speaker's languages, and in various structural relationships (i.e. positions within the syllable).
2. The style portrayed should not only include differences such as formal v. informal, but also various degrees of code-switching (i.e. changing from L1 to L2 within an utterance, or set of utterances).

3. In the case of bilinguals, the situation criterion should not refer solely to tests as opposed to free conversation, but should include the ability of the assessor to interact in both (or all) the languages, so as to produce examples of L1, L2 and code-switching.

Mueller, Munro and Code (1981) describe two of the most widely-used articulation tests in detail: the Edinburgh Articulation Test – EAT (Anthony *et al.*, 1971), and the Goldman Fristoe Test of Articulation – GFTA (Goldman and Fristoe, 1972), as well as discussing a phonological processes approach (though not in terms of any standardised procedure).

In their discussion of the EAT, Mueller *et al.* point out several advantages in this test, for example the quantitative section, where points given to various responses can provide an overall score from which it can be seen whether the subject is above or below a *danger level* in relation to normal phonological acquisition. A qualitative assessment is also undertaken which does aid in the discovery of patterns of phonological change affecting similar classes of sounds. However the test is still criticised in their overall appraisal. For example, in the qualitative assessment it is not always clear how to classify errors; furthermore neither of the two sections provide guidance as to therapeutic strategies, and overall 'the EAT . . . provides little direct information on the child's ability to use sounds to signal differences in meaning' (Mueller *et al.*, 1981, p. 22).

The GFTA is similar in concept to the EAT, but has a slightly different make-up. Sounds are tested in words (as in the EAT), in sentences through the retelling of a story, and finally any mispronounced sounds are retested in an imitation procedure. Throughout, the transcription of the individual target phonemes is required, not the whole word. A score is calculated from the first two sections.

Mueller *et al.*, criticise the test mainly because of the phoneme-in-position approach, which will obscure broader patterns and word-structure effects. This is particularly unfortunate as the story section, if fully transcribed, would have provided much useful data in this area. Although the final section (imitation practice) is helpful, overall the authors feel 'this test could be said to provide phonetic information . . . but it is not able to provide a real insight into the phonological patterning of child speech' (Mueller *et al.*, 1981, p. 26).

The authors' description of a phonological process approach is not restricted to a particular procedure, as these are only just being devised (see Grunwell, 1982; Crystal, 1982). The appraisal of this type of approach reflects much of what was said concerning natural phonology above. The main advantages being that 'it has the potential to explain what initially may appear to be random errors' (Mueller *et al.*, 1981, p. 31) and helps in the planning of therapy. This can be achieved through the comparison of the processes used by a patient with the normal developmental pattern. If, for example normal processes are persisting, it will be clear which of these normal processes are the most delayed, requiring treatment before another less delayed process. A process approach also leads to therapeutic strategies based on classes of sounds, rather than work on individual phonemes.

What of the assessment of the phonological proficiency of bilinguals? Abudarham (1979) points out that there are no standardised tests currently available that allow 'an individual to respond in either of . . . two languages, from a possible "bilingual" repertoire' (p. 232). This leads to the practice of testing via one language only – often not the speaker's dominant language.[2] As Abudarham (1979) notes, the use of standardised monolingual assessment procedures with bilinguals is 'of little, if any, diagnostic or prognostic value in the speech therapy clinic' (p. 232). Ball and Munro (1981) state 'many therapists are forced to make their own translations of English tests, while admitting this is by no means an ideal situation' (p. 232).

One answer that can be proposed to overcome this problem lies in the design of phonological assessment procedures for other languages, specifically those often found in bilingual situations in the country in question. Such a procedure for Welsh is described in Ball and Munro (1981). Such assessments, though useful, do not completely assess the *bilingual* nature of the phonology. (See the criteria noted above.)

Abudarham (1976, 1979, 1980) discusses how such a bilingual assessment could be designed in the specific area of vocabulary assessment. He feels that if many bilinguals can be considered as possessing, in functional terms, a single linguistic system, a test can be designed prompting words equally familiar in both languages, so that either can be used in response, and score as equally correct.

This sort of approach unfortunately is not directly applicable to the problems of phonology. As previously noted, the present standardised tests are criticised for lack of representativeness – a test of the sort which could accept either language as an answer would be even less likely to produce a representative sample of the system and structure of either language, let alone both – particularly where there are considerable differences between the two phonologies.

The solution proposed to these problems in monolingual assessments, the use of recordings of longer stretches of speech as well as or instead of elicitation tests, seems the answer also in the bilingual situation. It is of course feasible to devise an elicitation test, some of whose responses are designed to produce L1, others L2. It would, however, be long, unwieldy (it would be difficult to guarantee the child would use a particular language), and in effect would simply be two monolingual assessments put together. (See the discussion above on adequate data.)

The use of recorded stretches of speech can of course be criticised as being time-consuming; but as other assessment procedures (Crystal, Fletcher and Garman, 1976; Crystal, 1982) also require such recordings, common data bases can be set up for various assessments.

The data once collected can be analysed in terms of phonological processes – and these in turn plotted against a normal developmental profile, as suggested in many recent linguistic assessments (e.g. Ingram, 1976; Crystal, Fletcher and Garman, 1976; Crystal, 1982; Grunwell, 1982). This results in an assessment that compares the subject's phonological patterns with those of normal development for the particular age level in question, but most importantly the comparison should be with the normal development of the bilingual, not monolingual.

To achieve this requires data on the normal development of the languages in question in bilingual speakers. (Normal development of the two languages separately will not of course be adequate.) The establishment of phonological assessment procedures for bilinguals will require then much work, and indeed some might even say it is impossible due to the wide variety of dominance patterns, and the difficulty in finding categories from a continuum.

Interpreting Results

It should be recognised that whatever approach is made to phonological assessment, problems arise in the interpretation of the data required. In an error analysis procedure it is often difficult to decide which category an error should be assigned to, and Grunwell (1982) discusses some examples of these. If a phonological processes approach is adopted, it can be unclear whether a particular process should be classified as a persisting normal process or an unusual/idiosyncratic process. In other words, how often does a process have to be found in various subjects to count as 'usual'?

However, these problems are not the most important when working within the bilingual situation. We have already discussed potential differences between the monolingual's and the bilingual's acquisition of phonology; we must also examine the effects these may have on the interpretation of results. For example, in a bilingual Welsh-English child should the use of [k] for the Welsh sound /x/ be considered to be part of a persisting normal process affecting fricatives (e.g. fricative stopping), or is it interference from English which lacks /x/ from its phoneme inventory? Evidence from other fricatives could be of help here, but even so it could be difficult in this instance to distinguish between delay and interference. In problematical cases such as this it is obviously essential that whoever is undertaking the assessment is thoroughly aware of the normal phonological processes found in acquisition, and the system and structure of the phonologies being acquired. In the instance cited, if all the fricatives were replaced by stops, this would resolve the problem regarding /x/. If on the other hand only /x/ were affected, it would probably imply an interference feature, though it could be that /x/ just happens to be the last fricative to be 'freed' from this particular process. This uncertainty could be cleared up if adequate records existed of previous developmental patterns for the particular subejct, which might show for example that recently other fricatives had also been subject to stopping. Finally, the knowledge of which language constitutes the primary system, and which the secondary (discussed above) also helps in deciding problem cases: interference being more likely in the secondary system.

Phonological interference of the sort found in bilinguals, as opposed to second-language learners, is discussed in Baetens-Beardsmore (1982), who describes four main types of segmental interference. First, he notes *underdifferentiation* of phonemes where two phonemes of one phonological system are realised as one phoneme due to the influence of the second system. A case in point is that of certain Welsh-speakers in Patagonia who merge the distinction between /s/ and /ʃ/ in Welsh to a single phoneme /s/ under the influence of Spanish (see R.O. Jones, 1983). Baetens-Beardsmore (1982) gives as another example French-English bilinguals merging the English phonemes /i/ and /ɪ/.

A second type is *overdifferentiation* of phonemes. This involves a distinction present in one system being carried over unnecessarily into the second system. An example of phonemic vowel length from Schwyzertütsch being used in Romansch is given by Baetens-Beardsmore (1982, p. 61).

These first two categories have involved phonemic interference. Interference can of course also be present at the phonetic level. *Reinterpretation* occurs when 'the bilingual distinguishes phonemes of the secondary system by features which are relevant to the primary system but redundant in the secondary system' (Baetens-Beardsmore, 1982, p. 61). The example is given of Italian/English-speakers using geminate or double consonants when speaking English.

Finally, *phone substitution* may occur. Here both systems contain equivalent phonemes which are considered by the speakers as such, but the phonetic realisation of the primary system is used also in the secondary system. Another example from Patagonian Welsh can be given: initial voiceless plosives in Welsh are strongly aspirated, whereas aspiration is absent in Spanish initial voiceless plosives. Spanish-Welsh bilinguals often show phone substitution whereby the plosives in Welsh are realised as unaspirated (R.O. Jones, 1983).

It is pointed out by Baetens-Beardsmore (1982), following Weinreich (1953) and Haugen (1954), that interference is most likely to take place between similar sounds: 'greater similarity creates a greater likelihood of interference than does dissimilarity' (p. 61).

Apart from segmental interference, interference at the suprasegmental level is particularly common. This can affect stress and intonation patterns, but unfortunately little work seems to have been done in this area. Baetens-Beardsmore (1982) discusses some examples from Dutch-French bilinguals (pp. 62-3).

In instances where a bilingual speaks languages which are geographically in contact (Welsh-English, Dutch-French in Belgium, etc.), these features of interference can become established as the 'Welsh accent of English' or the 'Brussels accent of French', and such *residual interference* must not be interpreted as being part of an individual speaker's interference pattern. This implies that the phonological patterns of the L1 and the L2 should be examined as they are actually spoken in the environment in question, rather than choosing standard forms.

It should also be noted that interference can be viewed developmentally and statically (i.e. as a feature of adult speech). Although the above-mentioned interference features may be found in both phonological acquisition and in adult sound systems, there is of course a difference between the two situations. Whereas adult interference patterns tend to remain fairly static, children's patterns are much more likely to change. For example, a child being raised as a Welsh-English bilingual may have a primary Welsh system, in the preschool period, therefore perhaps showing interference in the secondary, English system. If that child then attends an English medium school, or even a bilingual school where the majority are English L1 speakers, the effects of peer group influence may cause a reversal of the primary and secondary systems, so affecting patterns of interference. As an example of this can be quoted data from a North Wales boy who in the pre-school period showed interference in English – most obviously the lack of the voiced fricative, [z]. After attending school in an English dominant area for several years, the interference was reversed – [z] was established in English, and his Welsh showed marked vowel quality changes, directly attributable to English.

The interference patterns of the second-language learner (rather than the bilingual) are usually similar in type to those outlined above, but can be much grosser thereby causing greater difficulty in comprehension.[3] Some of the most common problems experienced by learners of English as a second language are described in detail by O'Connor (1967).

It is clear therefore that in assessing a bilingual's phonology due attention must be paid to possible interference patterns, as being a phenomenon distinct from a phonological disorder.

Implications for the Clinic

The clinician wishing to assess a patient's phonology has a set of standardised tests to choose from, various theoretical models for analysing data, and with many languages, developmental norms for comparison. Whatever the shortcomings of the tests as noted above, it is possible to gain a good perspective of a monolingual's phonological abilities.

For bilinguals the position is quite different. We have discussed how assessment is often restricted to one language, or at the best to the two phonologies as quite separate systems; how minority languages (often L1 in minority bilingual communities) have very little language assessment material available.

The way forward in terms of assessing a bilingual's phonology lies through proper preparation and research. Whatever form of elicitation procedure is devised, however it is ensured that more or less equal amounts of L1 and L2 are recorded, the main problem lies in the analysis of the data. Normative information is essential before any adequate analysis of disordered phonology is feasible. Not only must the clinician have access to what is a developmental norm for the two languages, but information on typical interference patterns, or patterns of separate phonological development between the languages, must be available.

Such information takes time to gather, and of course the vast number of possible permutations of two languages (not to mention three or more) that a blingual speaker might be acquiring tend to suggest it is an impossible task. However, the more common combinations can be identified (in Britain the work of the Linguistic Minorities Project has done this; see for example Saifullah-Khan, 1980) and it is to be hoped that work on these will be forthcoming. Until then any assessment on a monolingual basis will be inadequate, and intervention strategies planned from such results will not be principled, and could well fail. Therapy linked to a process approach appears the most suitable answer, and although it may be a long time until full developmental details are available for bilinguals, what we know at present suggests that processes are not markedly different across language boundaries. We are therefore justified in supporting this approach as a basis for the assessment of the phonologies of bilinguals.

I would like to thank Siân Munro and Nik Miller for their helpful comments on earlier drafts of this section.

Notes

1. Such simultaneous acquisition is often considered as capable of producing speakers with a single 'compound' or 'fused' system. For further discussion of this and other classifications of bilingual acquisition see Abudarham (1980a).
2. For discussion of the measurement of language dominance see Baetens-Beardsmore (1982), Chapter 3.
3. It should be noted that the modern trend in second-language learning research is to equate errors with language-learning principles, rather than simply a straightforward interference.

7 ISSUES OF ASSESSMENT OF LIMITED-ENGLISH-PROFICIENT STUDENTS AND OF TRULY DISABLED IN THE UNITED STATES

Eva Gavillán-Torres

Introduction

The process of assessing limited-English-proficient (LEP) students in the United States and of determining which of those children are truly handicapped is a challenging task which encloses several problems.

The first problem is determining when a bilingual or monolingual (i.e. non-English-speaking) child has communication and learning problems due to his/her inability to perform in the English language. The second problem is determining which assessment tools are adequately designed to measure bilingual or monolingual children's language. The third problem is identifying assessment tools that can help teachers and evaluators determine a second-language acquisition problem from a real handicap.

This chapter will deal with these three problems from the perspective of a bilingual educator interested in the development of academic interdisciplinary programmes in bilingual-bicultural and special education. The chapter discusses the problem of assessment of LEP students who are suspected of having a handicap and have been labelled as mentally retarded (MR), learning disabled (LD), speech impaired (SI) or hearing impaired (HI).

Examples from Hispanic children will be used to illustrate some of the problems faced by LEP students who are suspected of having a handicap. Further, this group comprises the largest American ethnolinguistic minority population.

US Educational Policy for Handicapped and LEP Students

Public Law 94-142, the Education for All Handicapped Children Act (1975), is one of the most complete legislative pieces in favour of the educational rights of handicapped citizens in the world. Its contents take into account all the factors affecting the educational equity of handicapped children: the parents, the school and the service providers. The law acknowledges the culturally and linguistically different handicapped individual and states that these persons ought to be tested with tools in the language they understand best. Further, the law calls for interpreters of language for the child's parents during interviews for their Individualised Educational Plan.

Another important policy affecting linguistic minority children with or without handicaps is that of the Bilingual Education Act of 1967. In this legislation the language assessment of bilingual or non-English-speaking children is not exclusive to bilingual programmes but to *all* schools in the US. Thus there is a national policy for the assessment of LEP students (Silverman *et al.*, 1977).

Other significant policies or regulations pro-rights of LEP and handicapped citizens are Section 504 of the Rehabilitation Act (1973) and the Lau Remedies (1974). This last one is the result of court litigation for the correct educational placement of students whose primary language is not English. Court records contain significant judicial decisions in favour of the civil rights of LEP citizens, e.g. *Larry P.* v. *Riles*; *Diana* v. *State of California*; *Dyrcia* v. *New York City Board of Education.*

All of these court cases and regulations recognise sociocultural factors as crucial determinants in the education of LEP handicapped citizens. Further, they recognise that quality public education is vital to improve their opportunities for independent living.

An appropriate education for the LEP child suspected of handicaps will have to meet the unique needs of this child. Therefore, special education for many LEP children will not be the total educational approach. In addition to the special services, other bilingual services are basic to the child's experience. The previously mentioned legal resolutions advocate compatibility between the LEP handicapped learner and the school.

This chapter addresses the question of compatibility through a review of the issues on assessment and instruments used with LEP Hipsanic children suspected of having handicaps. The chapter has been divided into four sections:

1. Review of existing testing tools and placement procedures.
2. Issues on bilingualism and bidialectism and their relationship to remedial language placement procedures.
3. Alternatives to existing placement practices.
4. Conclusions.[1]

Additionally, two appendices are provided which include: a partial list of tests for Spanish-speakers and a select bibliography of works related to the assessment of LEP handicapped children not mentioned in the main text.

Review of Existing Testing Tools and Placement Procedures

There are important questions regarding the validity of many procedures used to identify and diagnose a handicap. In addition, there are some controversial issues in the design, development and administration of language sections of several psychological tests. Children who are limited-English-proficient (LEP) and those who speak other dialects may not respond to verbal sections of a standardised test because they have difficulty in recognising 'Standard English'. Thus there is the ever present possibility of misjudging the responses of minority group children. While educators have found alternatives to this problem in teaching (bilingualism, bidialectism), test developers have not acknowledged these differences, and consequently the risks of misplacement due to language and cultural differences continues to be very high (Adler, 1981). Both of these issues are dealt with in the following literature review. The literature review also discusses how existing testing procedures, even those with consideration to linguistic and culturally different children, are not helpful to teachers and students in their teaching and learning practices.

The list below includes the names of popular commercial tests used with Hispanic LEP children to determine: mental ability, achievement, speech and language (development, articulation and perception) and of some bilingual tools frequently used to determine the Hispanic LEP child's proficiency in English and/or Spanish. The list was prepared from the suggestions of a small group of professionals, and from Compton's (1980) and Darley and Siegel's (1979) Spanish tests selection. Thirty-four commercial tools were chosen as representative of what is commonly used and listed by specialist's area: i.e. mental ability, achievement, speech/language, bilingual (English/Spanish).

Mental Ability

1. Leiter International Performance Scale – Arthur Adaptation
2. Wechsler Intelligence Scale for Children – Revised
3. Slosson Intelligence Test
4. Bender Visual Motor Gestalt
5. Otis Lennon Mental Ability Test
6. Stanford-Binet Intelligence Scale

7. Henmon-Nelson Tests of Mental Ability
8. Pictorial Test of Intelligence
9. Culture Fair Series (Cattell)
10. Peabody Picture Vocabulary Test
11. System of Multicultural-Pluralistic Assessment
12. Goodenough-Harris Drawing Test

Achievement

13. Iowa Test of Basic Skills
14. California Achievement Test
15. Test of Basic Experience 2
16. Boehm Test of Basic Concepts
17. Metropolitan Achievement Tests
18. Stanford Achievement Tests
19. Wide Range Achievement Tests

Speech/Language

Development

20. Screening Test for Auditory Comprehension of Language
21. Test for Auditory Comprehension of Language
22. Del Rio Language Screening Test
23. Preschool Language Scales
24. Toronto Tests of Receptive Vocabulary
25. Spanish Accent Auditory Discrimination Test

Articulation

26. Austin Spanish Articulation Test
27. Southwestern Spanish Articulation Test
28. Denver Articulation Screening Examination

Perception

29. Illinois Test of Psycholinguistic Abilities

Bilingual (English/Spanish)

30. Basic Inventory of Natural Language
31. Bilingual Syntax Measure
32. Language Assessment Battery
33. James Language Dominance
34. Screening Test of Spanish Grammar

Problems in Tests Used with Hispanic LEP Children

Recent studies (1975-80) regarding the influence of tests on the learner have been accomplished in the social sciences field. It has been recognised that there are social and cultural influences on an individual's performance on a test. Social scientists have also considered the impact of labelling in particular handicapped children from cultural and linguistically different groups (Mercer, 1976). These two points are obviously related and are central to this chapter.

Diamond (1981), explains that bias in testing has been an issue of controversy over the past decade. Different procedures to detect bias have been used. For example: (1) editorial reviewers and reviews made by members of the groups to whom the bias is addressed; (2) psychometric and/or statistical methods to determine point estimates of bias, e.g. transformed p-values, transformed deltas, Rasch, chi-square (pp. 1-5).

The question is: are tests valid for the purposes for which they were intended when used with minority group children? The task of ensuring justice towards the different groups that are tested is what social scientists and some psychologists are questioning. The utilisation of tests that maintain sexual, racial and linguistic stereotypes is common practice and the primary cause of educational inequality.

Diamond also reports on the appropriateness of 'culture-free', 'culture-fair' and 'culture-specific' tools. These tests have been found to reflect only a small portion of a child's abilities and exclude many of the more important abilities needed by all children to succeed in school. The panel review and psychometric and/or statistical measures previously described have been adopted by publishers in an effort to establish 'bias-free tools'. But most of these procedures focused on what has been called 'facial' bias, with particular attention to male v. female presentations in texts, non-sexist language and ethnic differences. Items with stereotypic implications may be replaced by items which were more sensitive to the concerns of the group (Diamond, 1981, pp. 13-14).

To date, the combination of judgemental and statistical review is the only known procedure that has been adopted by researchers and publishers to identify bias in tests. Court cases such as the ones described earlier and resulting legislation have had significant impact on the testing procedures used to assess Hispanic and other minority children. Many of these cases have disputed the validity of IQ testing and usefulness of all IQ tools. Despite litigation and legislation, professionals in the field continue to use commercial tools such as the ones presented in the list. It cannot be said that there is a single group of tools that psychologists and educators use to test Hispanic LEP students or LEP students suspected of handicaps in general. This is the situation because these professionals employ a number of standardised testing tools that according to *their experience* are useful. These tools are then combined with commercial bilingual assessment tools, and, often, locally-developed Spanish/English language-screening and placement tests. This process is often followed by an interview with the parents and sometimes by a set of informal observations of the child's interactions (in school, in their home; see Chapters 9 and 10).

The alternatives used by practitioners, to date, to resolve the problem of testing Hispanic LEP children, tend to support the practice of testing only to get an idea of where the child's problem lies, without labelling. In other words, testing is only meaningful to the Hispanic LEP child if it is used for purposes of correcting a learning problem.

Sociolinguistic Factors that Tend to Affect the Assessment of Hispanic LEP Handicapped Children

Communication disorders is the general label used to present problems and findings on language development of children with special needs. Recent studies in child language development have postulated the fundamental assumptions of language-learning. A description of these assumptions and findings is reported by Bloom and Lahey (1978). They clarify these assumptions and findings by stating that language is a vehicle for messaging. Children with language development problems must get help in learning how language encodes their environment. As a child learns the elements for encoding he/she also learns the elements for messaging. Further, all language usage is social and embedded in culture. Thus, through language children learn to keep in communication with their environs (p. viii).

Research on the function of language has disclosed the importance of social influences on language, such as communication interactions needed between a speaker and listener in a given context. The circumstances involving the communication acts have influence on the language used; the relationship of the speakers and the content of messages will vary in each situation (Bloom and Lahey, 1978; Cook-Gumperz and Corsaro, 1975).

In summary, language is composed of content, form and use. Children acquire language 'naturally' in their homes and communities, with parents, relatives and peers. If we wish to describe children's language-learning processes, we must observe children's behaviours in different settings (e.g. home, play, school).

In light of the above discussion on language development it can be understood that the social functions of language are subject to culture. There are dialectal differences in language due to the influence of geography and location, socio-economic status, education and degrees of acculturation into the dominant ethnocultural groups. It is interesting that what prevails as dominant in one geographical area might be insignificant to other geographical areas from a social point of view (Adler, 1981). Dialect is the general label used to describe regional/geographical and social variety. In the US, dialect differences involve pronunciation and grammar as well as vocabulary differences of educated and undereducated groups. There is a direct relationship or connection between dialect, socio-economic status and place of residence. A child's sociocultural environment will affect directly his/her language acquisition. The child will imitate use and available speech in models (Adler, 1981, p. 36).

Issues on Bilingualism and Bidialectism and Their Relationship to Remedial Language Placement Procedures

This chapter suggests that the notion of a bidialectal and bicultural approach to educating Hispanic LEP children, with or without special needs, is basic to the children's optimal functioning abilities in school. This same argument has been proposed by Adler (1981) on behalf of poverty-stricken children. He suggests that a bidialectal and bicultural approach be utilised in conjunction with the conventional enrichment programme. This approach would insist on cultural practices in all educational and habilitative interactions with the child (p. x). Adler contends that poor children possess speech and language disorders in addition to their dialectal or linguistic differences (p. xii). For Adler, the educator and clinician of the poor must develop the ability to differentiate between communicative differences and deficits and communicative disorders and treat them accordingly. This can only be done if the clinician and educator are able to determine which speech patterns are deficient and which are not only different but also indicative of the specific population the child represents.

Bilingual educators recognise the fact that the education success of Hispanic LEP minority children will depend upon the opportunities they will receive through schooling to understand, hear and digest or assimilate the contents of the 'language used in the classroom', and the 'language used in tests'. Further, bilingual educators and researchers recognise that the language assessment tests used to determine the degree of bilingualism and handicappism in Hispanic and other LEP linguistic minority children are limited. Thus the process of documenting the language skills of these students is a central problem to the proper remedial placement of these students. However, bilingual educators and researchers continue to search for ways of documenting the language characteristics of these students; specifically those characteristics that can help them to distinguish between abnormal language development and delay problems.

A process being used frequently is the three-stage assessment methodology that includes (1) an oral language proficiency test, (2) teacher observations and ratings of their students' language abilities and (3) an ethnography of the child's language. In the first stage, commercial tests are used, some of which were listed previously in this chapter. In the second stage some form of standard observation scale is usally modified; widely used is Flanders Scale (1970) or any other scale listed in *Mirrors for Behavior II: An Anthology of Observational Instruments*, by Simon and Boyer (1970). Other home-made observations are also used. In the third stage of the process several procedures are used.

Erickson's (1981) ethnographic techniques use videotapes, cassettes or tapes of voice recorders and field notes to document interactions that occur in the classroom. Mace-Matluck, Hoover and Dominguez (1981) used taped samples of classroom situations to study variation in the use of Spanish-English, monolingual English and monolingual Spanish-speaking students. These researchers used cassette tape recorders and Lapel or Lavalier microphones to collect classroom language samples, and microcassette recorders to obtain home and playground samples. The latter was obtained by providing children with a specially designed belt/sash on which to put the portable recorder. In some instances the children would carry the recorders in their pockets (p. 4).

Carrasco (1979), Erickson (1981) and Cazden (1972), Duran (1981), Laosa (1977) and Santiago (1980) have used variations of the ethnographic approach in different bilingual settings and suggest this type of research is more sensitive to teacher and pupil dynamics. Further, this type of research reveals that Hispanic children are often viewed by their teachers as being 'naturally conditioned to failure' and also ignored because of language differences, abnormal behaviours in the classroom and even differences in physical appearance. The important thing is that this research approach provides for remedial and preventive actions, since the researcher can always ask the teacher and child to explain how they view each other in the classroom.

Erickson (1981) suggests that ethnographies of bilingual classrooms present research information that speaks for teaching and learning where both teacher and students adapt to the use of similar educational practices, such as the use of the child's primary language. This type of study helps the researcher identify situations where learning can be more effective and socially meaningful as it provides an index for immediate intervention.

The approach described above is most compatible with the latest sociolinguistic theories. In 1976, the Center for Applied Linguistics presented to the former Bureau of Education for the Handicapped a discussion on the contributions that sociolinguists could make to special education, specifically in the personnel preparation area.

Rudolph C. Troike, at that time director of the Center, presented an example from a child of a Portuguese family who had been labelled as emotionally disturbed. A linguist was called to provide additional assessment of the child's language disorders. The consultant utilised tapes to analyse the child's communicative patterns with school staff and peers. After gathering some data on the child's ethnocultural group, the linguistic consultant was able to produce a new set of evidence that challenged the child's educational placement in a programme for the handicapped (p. 2).

In light of the previous discussion it can be stated that any educational services for the LEP Hispanic child, in order to be appropriate, should be bilingual and bicultural. For all Hispanic children the bilingual services will be in two languages in terms of testing and in the interviews with parents or legal guardians. For Hispanic children with handicaps which prevent this type of learning, bilingual services will be a vehicle to increase their relatives' and community involvement in their rehabilitation and education.

It is a fact that there is a scarcity of tools to assess problems of delay, differences and deviation among LEP Hispanic children. Practitioners dealing with these children explain that there is need for alternate procedures to existing tests, that is, an approach to help the teacher and psychologist to get experience in identifying the particular needs of Hispanic handicapped children; an approach for determining handicaps in the Hispanic child with consideration to language and culture, i.e. a bilingual-bicultural approach.

Some practitioners explain that more than one standardised test is used in the assessment process and that roughly half of their Hispanic LEP students offered performance assessments come out with problems that can be resolved through conventional special education curriculums. The other half of their students' assessment is often too difficult to rely on tests alone. This half of the students cannot be described by known categories of physical dysfunction. Furthermore, these students cannot be referred and treated within the educational system.

Practitioners indicate that testers of Hispanic LEP students need extensive academic and practical experience on commercial testing tools and bilingual skills that respond to the child's language and its possible dialectal variations.

Early in this chapter it was stated that most of the commercial tools are lacking in their reliability and validity data. Further, the majority of tests have been developed based upon the medical design of abnormality versus normality. Cultural misconceptions of deviance have not been utilised in reanalysing those behaviours that were previously identified as 'abnormal'.

A pertinent example of a type of innovative study that can help to shed light on the kinds of interventions that are necessary to provide bilingual special education services is the Consortium for Hispanic Investigations in Language Development and Socialization (CHILDS) 1978. This group studied the socialisation process and its impact on communication ability through an analysis of the interaction between parents and children. The study consisted of observations over a two-year period in the family/home environment and involved categorising utterances in the socio/linguistic interactions between parents and children. Preliminary analysis of the data indicated that there are generational differences that affect the language environment of the Hispanic child. It was observed that first-generation language interactions occur in Spanish, third-generation occur in English. The study has identified some skill mastery communication patterns in adaptive, social, academic, cognitive, language and moral development skills that are considered a prerequisite for learning in a school setting. One area in which the study is very revealing is in the category of social and moral development skills, where the mother is more likely to control the social function/interaction of the child and uses specific language to express how those functions will happen. Mothers are most likely the ones who scold, and also the ones who teach the child the proper ways in accordance with the Hispanic culture (SSMHRC, 1978, pp. 7-8).

This type of sociolinguistic study provides information that can assist the special educator to implement language activities within the framework needed for proper language instruction of the Hispanic severe to profound child. The need for parent intervention programmes to incorporate the recommendations generated through these data will contribute to the development of effective curriculum approaches.

As a final point of illustration, an example from the speech and language profession will serve to present some trends and solutions in testing handicapped children. This professional area was chosen as Hispanic LEP students' handicaps, for the most part, are related to language usage.

Darley and Siegel (1979) explain that the primary focus of speech and language pathology has been in developing tests to determine auditory skills and auditory dysfunctions – problems in sound recognition and production, development and communication. Current theories of language development have had an effect on this field's approach to assessment (pp. iii-vi). More than thirty years ago, language was narrowly defined. Counting procedures, i.e. counting phonemes, utterances, their length, were used to diagnose language problems without consideration for psycholinguistic abilities. Current work in speech and language is influenced by Chomsky's work on the dimensions of language; its social and individual function and its developmental qualities. As such, new language tests focused on sentence production and are intended to measure the child's ability to understand a language and use its grammatical rules (pp. 1-3).

Other theories on language articulation and perception are still developing and many are controversial. Current theoretical work on language has not yet influenced language assessment for the Hispanic LEP student.

Professionals in educational research and measurement suggest that the mistakes made in educational assessment procedures may increase if educators begin to merge with those disciplines whose theoretical foundations were not formulated for education, e.g. interdisciplinary collaboration with medicine. If assessment is to serve to inform educational decisions then assessment procedures need to derive from psychological and educational theory, primarily, and only secondarily from other disciplines such as medicine. This should not be interpreted as meaning that culturally different children do not require proper medical attention, and that culture or education alone can take care of all their needs. However, the assumption underlying all educational assessment is that individuals, regardless of their disabilities or differences, can attain at least minimal education competency but that individualised methods of instruction are required to enable them to achieve prescribed goals (e.g. to brush his/her teeth; write his/her name; spell, other). The purpose of education assessment is to define appropriate educational goals and provide guidelines for individualised instruction.[2]

Since 1971 several innovative developments in speech and language disorders occurred which inspired the inclusion of new sources of knowledge (e.g. sociolinguistics) in the work of those people engaged in 'speech remediation' (M. Berry, 1980).

The Hispanic LEP child generates numerous concerns relative to the identification of speech problems that are truly a sign of a handicapping condition, and the speech patterns that reflect dual language acquisition or Spanish monolingual development. A description of the type of programme that is widely used in providing services to Hispanic LEP children in need of assistance in speech development falls in the category of 'enrichment programmes', because of assumed cultural, linguistic and/or economic disadvantages. In the discussion of this point, the reader will understand that some generalisations can be made in relation to a Hispanic LEP child's 'speech problem'. It is assumed that all children from culturally different backgrounds are deprived. The notion of cultural deprivation and disadvantage has been widely and – simultaneously – improperly used. Being different does not imply being disadvantaged or deprived. Problems of health due to poverty do not always translate into physical fragility. In fact, well-to-do children appear often to be as fragile as their poor counterparts both physically and emotionally. Adler, an expert in poverty-stricken children, contends that most problems with the children of the poor have to do with societal behaviours and rewards. In other words, Adler understands that there are several learning behaviours which respond to exclusive cultural patterns that are not represented by social institutions, and that do not allow students from other cultural groups to be adequately taught in the regular school environment (pp. 9-10).

For Hispanic LEP children and speakers of other dialects, it is important to recognise the role of their communicative mode or language in learning. This group of children are in need of professional assistance from individuals who understand the child's vernacular language and how it may not be compatible with traditional classroom instruction.

In the recent *Martin Luther King Jr. Elementary School Children et al.* v. *Ann Arbor School District Board* (1980) legal case, the need for incorporating the minority child's language in education was documented as the first step towards equal educational and social opportunity. This case maintained that failure of teachers to recognise and deal with minority children (in this case Black English speakers) caused many problems in a child's capacity to switch from vernacular English to standard English. This case challenged the educational system to retain educators and develop educational tools that recognise language diversity.

The tests listed in the previous section are the primary instruments used to evaluate a Hispanic LEP child suspected of having a handicap and language problems. It is important that assessment approaches and new tools be developed incorporating findings from current sociolinguistic research. For example the works of Fishman (1972), Gray (1978) and Cazden (1972) have been used by bilingual researchers to understand more about sociocultural influences on language development. The study of language use by different cultural groups and social classes has demonstrated that communication differences are not always representative of linguistic development problems.

Adler (1981) contends that speech teachers and testers have paid excessive attention to the way a child speaks and not to what he/she is saying (p. 109). This is a basic issue raised by bilingual educators regarding the evaluation of a Hispanic child who speaks the Spanish of his/her ethnic group. The issue here is not that Spanish-speakers from the different groups cannot communicate with each other; communication is possible and it takes place in everyday life of the Hispanic communities. Grammatically, every Spanish dialect is 'standard'. What we have here is a set of lexical choices that reflect indigenous influences of the various Hispanic groups. For example, Spanish from the Americas includes words representing Maya, Inca, Aztec, Taíno and European (not Spain) influence; words which represent different regions of the Spanish mainland and the Latin American nations; the phonological and pronunciation patterns which reflect geographical enclaves of Spanish speakers, e.g. coast, inland, other. Further, lexical terms are borrowed or extracted from such foreign languages as English and Romance languages (e.g. the Argentinian 'cocoliche'). There are also intonation or speaking styles which again represent geographical enclaves, e.g. Caribbean, Rio de la Plata, Frontier, other.

This should not be confused with speech defect. Nor should it lead to generalisations on the ability of Spanish-speakers to communicate with each other. However, it should be a source of training for those professionals who will deal with testing of this group. The example that follows is representative of one area of research and training for the speech and language professional working with Hispanic LEP children.

Syntactic and articulation deviations among Spanish-speakers have been studied extensively as demonstrated by the works of Canfield (1981). It can be said that some 'deviations' have gained such widespread acceptance among the members of various Hispanic groups, that they are considered to be 'normal language usage'. In 1976, Cancel conducted a research study investigating syntactic and articulation deviation among Spanish-speakers. Cancel speaks about the lisping behaviour in Spanish. He questions whether it is a language defect or dialectal trend. He explains how Spanish-speakers from the Caribbean islands' speech patterns differ from those of Central, South America and some parts of Spain (Cancel, 1976).

Their Spanish is not characterised by lisping but by distinctive regional pronunciation patterns. Two examples of these patterns are omission and aspiration of the /s/ sound and different patterns in the pronunciation of sibilant sounds. A conclusion derived from Cancel's study is that individuals should be assessed with respect to the individual's own vernacular language; and remediation, when appropriate, should be provided in the child's familiar language. If the child is learning English and appears to be proficient in this language the educator must consider that certain aspects of the child's more familiar language might interfere with or alter the pronunciation of certain words. For example, the Hispanic child might delete some consonantic sounds in English in the same way he/she deletes them in Spanish. The problem is a complex one and it is suggested that speech clinicians and educators who work with Hispanic LEP children receive special training in 'normal' ethnic speech patterns. Research conducted by Marcos *et al.* (1973) demonstrated how psychiatric patients (adults) of Hispanic descent were judged by experienced raters as exhibiting more psychopathological behaviours when interviewed in the English language than when they were interviewed in Spanish. Similar results occurred when interviewers integrated the use of English and Spanish. Patient conversations were marked by frequent misunderstandings, incomplete responses, stuttering, periods of silence and slowed speech. These behaviours are likely indicators of anxiety and depression (pp. 655-9). Similarly, when Hispanic children are interviewed in English, these children respond with withdrawal or silence. Many practitioners have determined that the lack of student cooperation during the interview process is a cue to emotional problems and disordered behaviours. It must be understood that knowledge of the language and culture alone, without awareness of normal and deviant behaviour patterns, is not enough to formulate an accurate and complete assessment of a speech language problem. It is important that the clinician and educator knows how to discern problems in both areas.

The ethnographic research approaches discussed in an earlier section of this chapter are becoming more important in understanding the learning behaviours of Hispanic LEP children. Knowledge of tests' limitations, particularly those imposed by language and culture, should also be acquired by the bilingual speech clinician. Therapeutic measures should be sensitive to the effect of environmental resources and support systems on language development. Finally, the cultural biases reflected by middle- and upper-class values should be re-examined in terms of teacher training and the curriculum available to minority students.

Alternatives to Existing Practices

The previous discussion indicates that there is no single standardised tool that can be considered as totally fair to Hispanic LEP students suspected of having a handicap. Therefore the use of these tests must be carefully supervised by professionals trained in their use and aware of the unique needs of these students. If the educator wants to differentiate between a Hispanic LEP child's language delay, difference or deviation problem he/she must rely on a variety of approaches such as the ones suggested earlier in this chapter. These approaches present a combination of strategies and devices, e.g. naturalistic language samples; tapes, records or videos of communicative interactions in the home, school, etc. and some type of grammatical analysis (e.g. Bilingual Syntax Measure, 1976).

In the case of the Hispanic LEP child the examiner, teacher and speech clinician must have command of the child's Spanish language with knowledge of the culture and its dialectal variations.

Bilingual-bicultural educators favour a multiprocess assessment procedure for children of LEP backgrounds. This procedure consists of: (1) observation (formal/informal); (2) interview (formal/informal); (3) testing; and (4) diagnostic teaching. Compton (1980) explains that this type of assessment contains all of the significant variables affecting the learning process of a child, for example, the home, the classroom, the school counsellor, other.

To date, no official guidelines have been developed to assist practitioners in determining what constitutes a delay, deviation or difference in the language of an Hispanic child. Most easily identifiable are the differences between the child's vernacular and its dialectal variations and the child's vernacular or dialect and English.

Promising sociolinguistic approaches such as the Language Assessment Remediation and Screening Procedures (LARSP) of Crystal *et al.* (1976) will have little impact on the LEP student until bilingual-bicultural special educators and researchers develop scales for each of the stages in bilingual language development. Before adapting the LARSP or similar approach we must find answers to questions such as:

- How can we represent bilingual language development accurately, i.e. in a scale?
- How many scales are needed to represent the subtleties in bilingual language development, e.g. vernacular scales or dialectal scales?
- How can we describe normal language development, i.e. by the child's vernacular and its usage patterns in the country of origin or by its usage patterns in the ethnic community?

Further, we must look into other types of influences and account for them in the development of new test measures. Significant issues to be raised are:

- What are the best criteria for determining normal language development, i.e. physiological, sociocultural, regional norms, ethnic norms, other?
- What is the impact of mass media in the environment of the LEP child and its language or communication mode?

Legislative efforts such as the ones described at the beginning of this chapter will remain incomplete until we have a cadre of highly specialised bilingual-bicultural/special educators and testers.

To alleviate the LEP student problems some short-term alternatives are:

- The development of bilingual-bicultural/special education resource centres to re-educate those teachers and professionals who are presently providing services.
- The development of a method for ascertaining the value of commercial tests by areas of handicap, for use with LEP children.
- The development of an international network to assist US researchers and educators in sharing information on test development

and norming and educational projects. This network could evolve into a clearing-house to disseminate adaptations and developments of new and existing commercial and/or privately developed tests in the world.

New approaches will come to light with the implementation of bilingual-bicultural special education. Conscientious experimentation is essential to the development of education programmes for the LEP student suspected of having a handicap.

Conclusions

The previous discussion fails to present an appropriate solution to the education of LEP handicapped students.

There are no simple answers or solutions to the language assessment and educational placement problems of LEP students suspected of handicapping conditions. At the present time very little is known about how to teach these students in classes for 'special children'. More research is needed in the area of behavioural differences of 'normally developed LEP students' and those who appear as delayed or deviant. These studies should shed light on the ways in which LEP children who are handicapped think and interact when compared to LEP children who are 'normal' or 'close to normal'.

An interdisciplinary agenda for research must be developed. Some sample questions to be included are:

- How do LEP handicapped students process information?
- Which environments are more appropriate for this process to take place?
- How do LEP handicapped students use language, i.e. in what situations?
- Can the learning problems of these students be separated by setting, i.e. school, home, play?
- When do these students function optimally?

If we continue studying the problems of LEP students in isolation, the answers to our research questions in the area of handicapping conditions will be vague. The interaction among the different disciplines that comprise bilingual-bicultural special education is most important to the development of meaningful and adequate learning programmes and services for the LEP handicapped group.

Time is running away and these children are suffering unnecessarily. We must start right now!

Notes

1. This chapter was prepared based upon a review of educational research literature conducted by the author under the sponsorship of the Rockefeller Foundation Minority Scholars Program (1981-2). This work included a thorough review of dissertations, journals, reports and other education related materials on the tests that are available to teachers and other education related professionals of Hispanic LEP children.

2. Once a Hispanic child is 'certified as ill', a problem arises which the medical approach alone cannot handle. The sole use of therapeutic instruction is not a sufficient means of handling the vast array of social and economic problems that these children face. The handicapped condition becomes the least of his/her problems. While unable to communicate, this child and his/her parents are not informed of their rights nor do they fully understand the many problems that affect them.

Appendix A Partial List of Tests for Spanish-speakers

Name	*Publisher*
Austin Spanish Articulation Test Elizabeth Carrow-Woolfolk	Teaching Resources Corporation 50 Pond Park Road Hingham, Massachusetts 02043 (617) 749-9461
Bilingual Syntax Measure M. Burt, H. Dulay, E. Hernandez	Harcourt Brace Jovanovich, Inc. Polk and Geary Streets San Francisco, California 94109
(Boehm Test of Basic Concepts) Ann E. Boehm Prueba Boehm de Conceptos Basicos	The Psychological Corporation 304 East 45th Street New York, New York 10017
Del Rio Language Screening Test Allen S. Toronto, D. Levermen, Cornelia Hanna, Peggy Rosenzweig, Antonieta Maldonado	National Education Laboratory P.O. Box 1003 Austin, Texas 78767

Name	*Publisher*
Developmental Assessment of Grammar Allen S. Toronto	Refer to: *Journal of Speech and Hearing Disorders*, 41, 2 (1976), pp. 150-71
Illinois Test of Psycholinguistic Abilities (Spanish Version)	Department of Special Education College of Education University of Arizona (602) 626-3214
James Language Dominance Peter James	Learning Concepts 2501 North Lamar Austin, Texas
Preschool Language Scale (Spanish Version) I.L. Zimmerman, V.G. Steiner, R.L. Evatt	Charles E. Merrill Publishing Co. 1300 Alum Creek Drive Box 508 Columbus, Ohio 43216
Screening Test for Auditory Comprehensive Language English/Spanish Elizabeth Carrow-Woolfolk	Teaching Resources Corporation 50 Pond Park Road Hingham, Massachusetts 02043 (617) 749-9461
Peabody Picture Vocabulary Test (Spanish Version)	American Guidance Service Publishers' Building Circle Pines, MN 55014
Screening Test of Spanish Grammar Allen S. Toronto	Northwestern University Press 1735 Benson Avenue Evanston, Illinois 60201
Southwest Spanish Articulation Test Allen S. Toronto	Academic Tests, Inc. P.O. Box 18613 Austin, Texas 78760
Test for Auditory Comprehension Language Elizabeth Carrow-Woolfolk	Learning Concepts 501 North Lamar Austin, Texas 78705

Name	*Publisher*
Toronto Tests of Receptive Vocabulary (English/Spanish)	Academic Tests, Inc. P.O. Box 18613 Austin, Texas 78760
Spanish Accent Auditory Discrimination Test	Peter Proul Merced County Department of Education 632 West 13th Street Merced, CA 95340

Appendix B Select Bibliography on Issues of Assessment and Placement of Limited English Proficient Children Suspected of Having a Handicap

DAI = Dissertation Abstracts International

A. General

Clarizio, H. (1979) 'SOMPA A Symposium Continued: Commentaries', *School Psychology Digest*, 8, 1

De Avila, E. and Havassy, B. (1974) *I.Q. Tests and Minority Children.* ED 109261

Dean, R. (1977) 'Brief Report on the WISC-R: V. Reliability of the WISC-R with Mexican-American Children', *J. of School Psychology*, 15, 3,267-8

Diamond, E. (1981) *Item Bias Issues: Background Problems, and Where We Are Today*, AERA, Los Angeles

Educational Testing Service (1980) ERIC Clearinghouse on Tests, Measurement and Evaluation, N.J., Highlights: *Culture-Free Tests*, January 80, and *Racial and Cultural Bias in Measurement Instruments*

Figueroa, R.A. (1979) 'The System of Multicultural Pluralistic Assessment', *School Psychology Digest*, 8, 1

Gavillán-Torres, E. (1980) 'An Interdisciplinary Approach to the Education of Hispanic Children', *Education Unlimited*, 2, 4, September/October

Goodman, J. (1979) 'Is Tissue the Issue? A Critique of SOMPA's

Models and Tests', *School Psychology Digest*, 8, 1

Laosa, L. (1977) 'Historical Antecedents and Current Issues in Non-discriminatory Assessment of Children's Abilities', *School Psychology Digest*, 6, 3, 48-56

Marmorale, A. and Brown, F. (1975) 'Comparison of Bender-Gestalt and WISC Correlations for Puerto Rican, White and Negro Children', *J. of Clinical Psychology*, 31, 3, 456-68

National Institute of Mental Health (1975) *Psychological Tests and Minorities*, Rockville, MD (R. Williams, Investigator)

Northeast Regional Resource Center (1980) *Task Force on Cross-cultural Assessment*, Hightstown, New Jersey

Padilla, A. (1979) 'Critical Factors in the Testing of Hispanic Americans: A Review and Some Suggestions for the Future', *Testing, Teaching and Learning*, NIE, Washington, DC

Shutt, D.L. and Hannon, T., *The Psychological Evaluation of Bilingual Pupils Utilizing the Hiskey-Nebraska Test of Learning Aptitudes, A Validation Study*, 12 ED 109215

Stewart, D. (1976) 'Effects of Sex and Ethnic Variables on the Profiles of the Illinois Test of Psycholinguistics and Wechsler Intelligence Scale for Children', Central Louisiana State Hospital, Pineville, *Psychological Reports*, February, 38, 1, 53-4

Swardlik, M. (1978) 'Comparison of WISC and WISC-R Scores of Referred Black, White, and Latino Children', *Journal of School Psychology*, 16, 2, 110-25

Vess, S. (1978) 'Testing Mexican American Primary Grade Children with the Human Figure Drawing and the Bender-Gestalt Test', *DAI*, University of Illinois, vol. 38 (10-A), 5978

B. Bilingual

Buell, K., Comp. and others (1973) *An Annotated List of Tests for Spanish Speakers*, ETS, Princeton, N.J., ERIC Doc. ED079393

Burt, M. and Dulay, H. (1978) 'Some Guidelines for the Assessment of Oral Language Proficiency and Dominance', *TESOL Quarterly*, 12, 2, 177-92, ERIC Doc. EJ181735

Carrasco, R.L. (1979) *Expanded Awareness of Student Performance: A Case Study in Applied Ethnographic Monitoring in a Bilingual Classroom*, SEDL, Austin TX

Educational Testing Service (1979) ERIC Clearinghouses on Tests, Measurements and Evaluation, N.J., Highlights: *Testing Spanish-Speaking Students, Testing Bilingual Students*

Ehrlich, A., Comp. (1973) *Tests in Spanish and Other Languages and*

Nonverbal Tests for Children in Bilingual Programs, CUNY, N.Y., Hunter College, Bilingual Education Applied Res. U., ERIC Dec. ED078713

Fiege, K. (1977) *Reading in a Second Language*, ED 144397

Finnocchiaro M. and King P.F. (no year) *Bilingual Readiness in Earliest School Years*, ED033248

Glass, L. (1979) 'Coping with the Bilingual Child', *AHSA*, p. 512, August

Gray, T. (1978) *Skills and Competencies Needed by the Bilingual-Bicultural Special Educator*, CAL, VA

Hilmer, S. (1977) *Demonstration of Assessment of Language Dominance of SpanishSpeaking Bilinguals. Occasional Papers on Linguistics*, no. 1, Southern Illinois University, Carbondale, April

Kuhlman, N. (1978) *Language Dominance Testing: Some Questions.* Paper presented at the annual meeting of the California Association of Teachers of English to Speakers of Other Languages, ERIC Doc. ED154614 (7th San Francisco, CA, March 3-5)

Locks, N.A. and others (1978) *Language Assessment Instruments for Limited English-Speaking Students: A Needs Analysis*, ERIC ED163062, NIE, Washington, DC, October

Matluck, J. and Mace, B.J. (1979) 'Language Characteristics of Mexican-American Children: Implications for Assessment', *J. of School Psychology*, 11, 4, 365-86

Nagy, L.B. (1972) *Effectiveness of Speech and Language Therapy as an Integral Part of the Educational Program for Bilingual Children*, DAI, United States International University, San Diego, California, vol. 33 (3-A), p. 1048, September

Pickering, M. (1976) 'Bilingual/Bicultural Education and the Speech Pathologist', *ASHA*, vol. 19, p. 275

Sanchez, R. (1976) 'Critique of Oral Language Assessment Instruments', *Journal of the National Association for Bilingual Education*, 1, 2, 120-7 Eric. Doc. EJ160855

Watson, B. and Van Etten, C. (1977) 'Bilingualism and Special Education', *Journal of Learning Disabilities*, 10, 6, 331-8

Zirkel, P. (1973) *A Method for Determining and Depicting Language Dominance*. Paper presented at the Annual Convention of Teachers of English to Speakers of Other Languages, ERIC Doc. ED086028

C. Mental Retardation

Baca, L. (1974) *A Survey of Testing, Labeling and Placement Procedures to Assign Mexican-American Students into Classes for*

Educable Mentally Retarded in the Southwest, DAI, University of Northern Colorado, p. 214, vol. 36/01-A

Gimon, A.T. (1973) *Maternal Expectancies: Effects of Their Modification on Training Behaviour of Puerto Rican Mothers Toward Their Retarded Children*, DAI, Yeshiva University, p. 6482, vol. 34/10-A

Hausman, R. (1972) *Efficacy of Three Learning Potential Assessment Procedures with Mexican-American Educable Mentally Retarded Children* DAI, George Peabody College for Teachers, 3438, vol. 33/07-A

Hoernicke, P. (1974) *The Morphological Development of Language in School Age Chicano Educable Mentally Retarded*, DAI, University of Northern Colorado, 2807, vol. 35/05-A

Ramos, E. (1978) *A Study of the Classification of Mexican-American Students as Educable Mentally Retarded Through the Use of Inappropriate Culturally Biased Intellectual Assessment and Procedures*, DAI, University of California, Irvine (vol. I, Test: vol. II: Appendix) vol. 39 (4-A) 2580-1

Suraci, A.B. (1967) *Reactions of Puerto Rican and Non-Puerto Rican Parents to Their Mentally Retarded Boys*, DAI, New York University, vol. 27 (11-A) 3739-40

Teller, H. (1975) *A Comparison of Levels of Retardation for Two Groups of Adolescents, Anglo and Hispanic, Using the Vineland Social Maturity Scale and the Wechsler Later Intelligence Scale for Children*, DAI, United States International University, San Diego, California, vol. 36 (5-B) 2455-6

Thomas, G.E. (1968) *A Comparison of Language Concept Development Among Spanish-American and Caucasian Average and Mentally Retarded Children*, DAI, Colorado State College, vol. 29 (4-A) 1055-6

8 READING AND THE BILINGUAL CHILD – ASSESSMENT AND REMEDIATION

Eleanor Anderson

At the outset it would seem sensible first to consider what is meant by reading and second to look closely at the nature of the reading process.

In order to participate fully in our society it is necessary to do more than accurately match spoken and written forms of the language; it is also necessary to understand what one reads and to be able to relate what is read to past, present and future experience. By reading, then, is meant thinking in the context of print. The reader should be actively engaged in interrogating the text, addressing the writer in terms of who he is, what his qualifications and experience are, why the passage was written in the first place, what its purpose is.

Having said that reading is thinking in the context of print, one might ask what is so special about print? Indeed, it is this 'specialness' of print that is at the root of many reading difficulties, and which by the same token may provide the basis for instruction in processing visual language. I shall return to this point, but for now let us look at the nature of the reading process.

The Reading Process

In decoding a text in English we have a number of sources of information available to us. These are briefly:

visual cues	the marks on the page
orthographic cues	the arrangement and grouping of letters
syntactic cues	the grammatical patterning of the text
semantic cues	the meaning of the text and the reader's previous knowledge of what is or is not likely to occur, including knowledge and understanding of the cultural context of what is read.

Although it is convenient in this context to separate out the cue systems, they clearly overlap and work together for the reader. The order in which they are presented is also one of convenience and in no way is intended to suggest either the acceptance of a 'bottom up' model of reading, where one builds up from the smaller units of language to the larger units of 'meaning', or a rejection of a 'top down' model of reading; it is intended to present an interactive model of reading where all the cue systems available may be used in any order and in any combination.

The assumptions being made then are that the reader has the perceptual, cognitive and linguistic knowledge and experience to make use of these systems. However, in a literate society we also assume that the reader wants to learn to read and sees sense and purpose in the activity. It is essential therefore that the materials used are worth reading and that the activity has some purpose. But skilled instruction and interesting materials of themselves are not enough. Reading should consist of a confident and active interrogation of the text, and this is certainly not likely to happen if the self-concept and cultural values of the learner are not preserved.

Types of Difficulties which Linguistically Competent Monolinguals may Experience in Learning to Read and Write

Using Visual Cues. The reader has to learn to respond to and discriminate between the shapes of individual letters, both in lower and upper case and in a number of typographical variations. Poor visual memory is a major cause of spelling difficulty. Both visual perception and visual memory may be assisted by exploring shape through tracing, drawing, writing and handling letter shapes. Poor motor control may slow down this process. Letter orientation may also create difficulties for readers in the early stages. They have learned that objects remain the same no matter how they are placed, but they then find that letters change according to their orientation, e.g. b, d, p, q. Reading and writing in English involves moving from left to right along the line and from top to bottom of the page.

Using Orthographic Cues. In order to make use of orthographic cues it is necessary normally to be able to discriminate between the phonemes of the language and then to match sound to written symbol. However, there are approximately 44 phonemes in English and only 26 letters and the relationship between them is by no means simple. Ability to discriminate between phonemes and to match with graphemes will be related to hearing and to willingness to listen and observe as well as experience of listening to spoken language and seeing written language. As written language differs from spoken language it is particularly important that those in the early stages of learning to read have as many opportunities as possible to listen to 'the language of books' being read aloud.

Using Syntactic Cues. If we were dependent on visual and orthographic cues alone, reading would be a much slower and more tedious business than it is. Our knowledge of the syntactic patterning of language enables us to sample from the text and predict with fair certainty the type of word or group of words that is likely to occur in a particular setting and thus require only a brief glance for confirmation. Lack of knowledge of this syntactic patterning or inability to apply such knowledge may slow down reading speed considerably and in turn put a larger load on memory.

Using Semantic Cues. Knowledge of semantics also enables the reader to predict and sample his/her way through a text. For example, in the following sentence, from a knowledge of syntax one would predict that the missing word is a noun:

The cat climbed up the ——.

From a knowledge of semantics, including knowledge of cats, the uncertainty of the missing word can be reduced to a handful of nouns such as: fence, tree, wall, curtains. It is only when one is very confident in the use of language that these bounds may be stretched to their limits for special purposes such as imagery or humour.

Lack of semantic knowledge or of ability to apply such knowledge has serious implications both for fluent reading and for comprehending what is written. This may occur through lack of background knowledge to provide a framework for understanding the text, or through insufficient knowledge or experience of the register employed, or through lack of understanding knowledge or experience of features of written texts that either do not occur in spoken language or occur in a different form.

Types of Difficulties that Second-language Learners, Literate in Their First Language, may Experience in Learning to Read and Write

Using Visual Cues. Confusion may well occur between the system of symbols used in the second language and systems in the first language with regard to letter formation, letter identification, position of symbols relative to horizontal lines on paper and directionality. For example, if Greek is the first language and English the second there may be confusion between the following letters:

Greek letter	*nearest English equivalent*
β	B
δ	d
ρ	p
αυ	au

For those accustomed to using Hindi script, letters are written below the line and in most cases the top of the letter touches the line so that the writing appears to be hung from the line, whereas for those used to reading or writing Urdu script, the direction is from right to left.

Using Orthographic Cues. There may also be confusion between phoneme grapheme correspondence in the first language and in the second language. In the Greek example just cited such a confusion might lead to misreadings such as:

English letter	*read as*	*on basis of Greek letter*
B	/v/	β
d	/ð/	δ
p	/r/	ρ
au	/av/	αυ

The most extreme forms may be between a first language that uses an ideographic writing system such as Chinese where generally a character stands for an object or an idea or an event, and a second language such as English that uses an alphabetic system with an irregular correspondence between grapheme and phoneme. An intermediate stage exists in Japan where Japanese children are taught to read using *hiragana*, a syllabary in which the correspondence between written and spoken syllables is very regular, and only when reading in *hiragana* is fluent do they transfer to reading *kanji*, the Chinese originated ideographic writing system.

Using Syntactic Cues. Difficulties in this respect may arise from two sources. The first is from inadequate knowledge of the syntax of the second language so that prediction and consequently fluency in reading are reduced and there is less opportunity to grasp the overall meaning of the passage as one proceeds. The second difficulty is from confusion between the syntax of the first language and that of the second. For example, in Vietnamese there are no separate forms for personal pronouns and adjectives. The meaning is determined by the word order. Similarly, the verb 'to be' is often omitted in Vietnamese and the Vietnamese-speaker may continue to do this when writing in English.

Using Semantic Cues. Difficulties in this area may be similar to those of monolinguals learning to read but deriving both from inadequate knowledge of the semantics of the second language and from confusion with the first language. Particular difficulties may arise when dealing with a range of registers, colloquialisms and text features beyond the sentence. Magda Leonardi (1981), from her experience of teaching Italian-speakers to read English, provides examples of difficulties that may occur with intersentential connectors. And Steffensen (1981) demonstrates how readers who share the cultural background of the writer 'come equipped' with the appropriate schemata to the task of comprehending text.

Types of Difficulties that Bilinguals Who are not yet Literate in Any Language may Experience in Learning to Read and Write

Using Visual Cues. In this case the learner may share all those difficulties encountered by the monolingual learner as well as some experienced by the bilingual already literate in one language.

Using Orthographic Cues. Once more the learner may experience all the difficulties of the monolingual learner. In addition, having access to the phonological systems of two languages, the number of options available to him/her in predicting phonemic patterns may be very much wider than for the monolingual learner, until the bilingual reader is able to separate consciously the two phonological systems.

Using Syntactic Cues. Similar confusions occur between the syntactic systems of the two languages as are experienced by the literate bilingual reader learning to read a second language.

Using Semantic Cues. All those difficulties which may be encountered by the monolingual learner and by the bilingual learner already literate in a first language may be experienced by the bilingual learner not yet literate in any language. Of particular importance, as has been indicated already, may be experiential and cultural differences which are not taken account of in the content of the reading material or in the expectations of the writer.

However, it would be only too easy to overemphasise the possibility of linguistic difficulties. There is no reason why bilinguals should find reading and writing in two languages necessarily any more difficult than monolinguals do in one language. For every difficulty one might suggest, there are many advantages. A high level of literacy in more than one language is an enormous advantage and an invaluable resource. What is important is that the teacher, therapist or psychologist is aware of and respects major linguistic and cultural differences and does not place unnecessary obstacles in the path of the learner. Indeed, as Moseley and Moseley (1977, pp. 66-7) point out in their review of research on language and reading among underachievers, there are significant gains in reading and language performance where home and school contacts are fostered.

Assessment and Description of These Difficulties with Particular Reference to the Differential Diagnosis Between a True Learning Difficulty and a Second Language Difficulty

Using Visual Cues. The most useful tests of perception related to literacy are those that make use of print, such as Marie Clay's *Concept of Print Tests: Sand and Stones* and *The Early Detection of Reading Difficulties: a Diagnostic Survey with Recovery Procedures.* Specific language difficulties may be identified by giving the test in two versions, one in each language. However, as the Goodmans (1982) have pointed out, it is not even necessary to use the original test booklet. It is possible to apply the questions to other books. But for work with bilinguals where there are considerable differences between the writing systems the original Clay test booklets would seem particularly useful.

Using Orthographic Cues. It is essential that children's hearing is checked. As Clark (1980) pointed out, minor hearing loss which is not significant in a clinical setting, may be crucial in a normal, busy classroom. High noise level does seem to be one of the school variables associated with poor reading performance (Moseley and Moseley, 1977, p. 67).

Phonological development should be assessed as already outlined. The Swansea Test of Phonic Skills (Williams, 1970) and a diagnostic spelling test such as that developed by Margaret Peters (1975) may also be of value.

Using Syntactic Cues. Syntactic development may be assessed as already outlined. The use of syntactic cues in reading may be assessed by a miscue analysis (Goodacre, 1979; Goodman and Goodman, 1977) in which the reader's miscues or errors in oral reading are considered in terms of syntactic acceptability. It is worthwhile to tape record the oral reading and transcribe and analyse it at a later date. It is essential that when carrying out a miscue analysis the teacher does not intervene in the reading but allows the reader to guess and to self-correct. After the oral reading the reader should be asked to recall as much as possible of the passage read so that some indication is given of the sense the reader made of the passage. Alternatively or additionally, cloze tests may be prepared with particular syntactic features deleted. The choice of deleted items and the interpretation of responses should take into account syntactic features that it is anticipated may cause particular difficulty, e.g. pronouns in the case of Vietnamese-speakers.

Using Semantic Cues. The procedure in this case is similar to that for the use of syntactic cues. Additionally, account should be taken of previous knowledge, otherwise scores on individual comprehension tests may overestimate or underestimate reading ability. It is occasionally worthwhile giving the questions on their own before the passage is presented and then asking the same questions at a later date after the passage has been read. The difference between scores provides an indication of the amount of information that has been gained from the texts.

In order to gain information about the effects of text structure and cultural setting some of the techniques employed by Steffensen (1981) in her research on cross-cultural reading comprehension might be adapted for classroom or clinic use. For example, passages from different cultural settings may be prepared in the following manner. The passage is presented in a booklet so that on each page one more clause is exposed than on the preceding page, with all the remaining clauses blanked out. Pupils then read the text a clause at a time and are asked to describe what they have already learned from the text and what they anticipate will follow.

Tasks that involve the sequencing and rearrangement of single sentences into a complete text also provide information on weaknesses in the perception of textual features that cross sentence boundaries. Both sets of activities may be carried out individually or in groups. Individual work provides more information for diagnosis but group work with an emphasis on discussion and justification is a particularly powerful teaching technique.

Guidelines and Suggestion for Remediation

General. It is rather obvious, but none the less necessary, to state that intervention must be based on accurate diagnosis first of language ability and second of reading ability. Language may be assessed as already outlined earlier in this book. It is essential to bear in mind differences between spoken and written language such as:

- Speech consists of sounds, while writing consists of visible marks. The sounds of spoken language are not heard as separate units, while in written language letters are represented as distinct shapes and words are separated by spaces.
- Spoken language occurs in time while writing occurs in space. Spoken language is generally less permanent than writing. Writing can be used to assist memory. Written language 'preserves a message through time' and as Donaldson and Reid (1982, p. 7) continue 'being able to put our thoughts on paper makes it possible to reflect, to edit, to revise, to restructure, and to take time'.
- On the whole speech is social whereas writing is generally solitary, with the writer and the reader separate from each other. This means that in reading the extralinguistic cues of facial expression and gesture are missing as well as cues such as intonation, rhythm and stress and the opportunity in a face-to-face setting of questioning and asking for further explanation or examples.
- Spoken and written language may also differ both in vocabulary and grammar and in the situations and purposes for which they are used. Finally, in writing and reading we are normally removed from the objects and situation to which the language refers.

These points are taken from Mackay, Thompson and Schaub (1970, pp. 112-27) where they are dealt with at greater length and in a particularly clear and useful manner.

As well as remembering the differences between the abilities required to deal with spoken and written language, it is also important to remember that reading difficulties may emerge at all levels. Some linguistic difficulties become apparent only in linguistically and conceptually difficult texts where the reader does not have a great deal of background knowledge (V. Edwards, 1980; Anderson, 1979). For those with an interest in and concern for language, it is easy to forget that 'language is simply one among a number of systems of meaning that are the property that constitutes human culture' as Halliday and Hasan point out (1980, p. 5), and in so doing to overestimate language ability from unsystematic and informal observation alone. However, the reader has to depend mainly on the linguistic system of meaning. Carpenter and Just (1977, p. 231) make the point very clearly when they state:

> The speaker can appeal to the perceptual context to supply information for the listener's discourse pointer and thereby make assumptions about the shared contextual information. In written discourse the writer and reader are removed in time and space so the pointer must be controlled almost entirely through the devices of language itself.

So the pupil who appears to cope well with oral language in a group setting may be responding well to non-linguistic communication cues and may well have quite serious problems of comprehension when reading demanding material on her/his own.

Specific Remediation of Difficulties in Using Visual Cues. There are many activities, approaches and materials used for reading readiness that may be adapted to the needs, interests and experience of the individual learner. In this respect the work of Clay (1981b) is particularly helpful as is that of Downing and Thackray (1975) and E. Hunter (1977). The Breakthrough to Literacy approach (Mackay *et al.*, 1970) provides a theoretically sound and practical overall approach.

The importance for the learner of hearing written language read aloud cannot be overemphasised. In the early stages it makes more sense for the teacher to read to the pupil from a shared book than vice versa. The learner's attention can be drawn in a natural and enjoyable manner to the relevant characteristics of print and to directionality. However, to do this the materials must be sufficiently interesting and motivating to support enthusiastic reading and re-reading until the learner begins to take over part of the task of reading. If numbers are too large to see the text that is being read then overhead projector slides, film strip or Language Master may be employed. For group or individual work tape/slide sequences, audio tapes alongside favourite books or the excellent BBC Listening and Reading series which involves tapes and books may be used. Awareness and understanding of a writing system develops rapidly through attempting to use it. Writing one's own name in it is an obvious starting point. But for fluent writing to be acquired it is essential that the writer is aware of the starting points for the formation of all letters and the direction in which they are formed. An easy, well-formed handwriting style assists spelling and writing in general (Peters, 1967).

Remediation of Difficulties in Using Orthographic Cues. There is a great deal of useful material available to assist with remediation in this area and those are listed in Raban (1980) and P. Edwards (1978). However the following reservations should be borne in mind when using them. First, remediation should be based on sound diagnosis and on perceived difficulties.

Secondly, what is taught should have a firm theoretical base. For further information on the orthographic patterning of English see Mackay *et al.* (1970), Albrow (1972), and Venezky (1976).

Practice should not consist of dull drills. There are plenty of games available, both in the form of suggestions for home-made versions and commercially produced games such as Stott's Programmed Reading Kit. There are numerous humorous books from those in the Language in Action series (Morris 1974) to the Dr Seuss books and collections of traditional rhymes.

The use of phonic cues should not be overemphasised to the detriment of the use of other cue systems. From the very beginning the emphasis should be on making sense of what is read and the expectation should be built up that what is read does make sense.

It should be remembered that ability to read aloud fluently is not necessarily accompanied by understanding of what is read. This may well be a particular problem for those already literate in one language who may find it relatively easy to learn the phonic rules for another language and this facility may encourage the teacher to overestimate her/ his ability.

Remediation of Difficulties in Using Syntactic Cues. It is important that the use of syntactic cues is encouraged from the earliest stages in reading instruction. In order to encourage this, to build up confidence and to provide content that is of interest and culturally relevant, a language experience approach may be employed. In this case the first reading material encountered is that which has been dictated by the learner and written down by the teacher. So the vocabulary, syntax and content are already familiar and the reader may make use of all the cue systems while she/he predicts her/his way through the text. This approach depends upon some familiarity with the spoken language and experiences about which to write. Robinson and Pehrsson (in press) provide some suggestions for work with pupils who are not sufficiently familiar with a language to make use of a language experience approach to reading. And Walker (1974) describes the use of such an approach with older pupils.

Penguin *Roll-a-Story* and *Find a Story* materials provide a great deal of amusing practice in simple sentence forms. They can be used individually, in pairs or in small groups. They are more fun to use when there is someone else there to share the fun.

Another approach to encourage attention to syntactic cues is to make use of a cloze procedure where particular syntactic items are deleted from a passage and the reader has to supply the missing words or acceptable alternatives. This may be done either as an individual acitivity which may be used for diagnosis and individual remedial work or as a group discussion activity where choice of word has to be justified and defended to the rest of the group. A similar approach dealing specifically with connectives is recommended by Leonardi (1981). As she points out, difficulties may arise because connectives do not necessarily translate directly from one language to another. This is not surprising when one considers that Gardner (1978, p. 27), in a study of logical connectives in science textbooks in Australia, found that 'most junior secondary school students have learned to employ "therefore" in a grammatically correct manner, but many have not learned to avoid using the term in logically unsound ways'.

Remediation of Difficulties in Using Semantic Cues. With the discussion of connectives the subject of semantic cues has already been broached. Although the remediation of difficulties in using semantic cues is a vital aspect of reading, it is also one which until recently has received little attention. The most promising lines for development would seem to be those identified by Pearson and Johnson (1978), Lunzer and Gardner (1979), Fitzpatrick (1981) and L.J. Chapman (1982). Pearson and Johnson are concerned with comprehension and the construction of questions; Lunzer and Gardner consider the use of group reading and discussion techniques; Fitzpatrick summarises possible areas of difficulty in classroom language of particular concern to bilinguals; and Chapman looks at the role of the perception of cohesion in the development of fluent reading.

In a recent review of bilingual education Lewis (1981) stated that 'Basic to the satisfaction of the needs of bilingual children appears to be sound and continuous instruction in language.'

There would be few who would deny this, but with the instruction must go respect for all of the learner's languages and close cooperation with his/her family. After all, Tizard *et al.* (1982) reported gains in the reading ability of children whose parents were encouraged to hear them read at home. This was regardless of whether the parents could read English or not.

Part 3

REMEDIATION

9 THE CASE HISTORY IN A CROSS-CULTURAL MILIEU

Niklas Miller

Part of the clinician's or teacher's task in the holistic approach to child assessment involves a general case history taking to place the child and his possible disorder in his contemporary and developmental context. Information from this procedure seeks to establish aetiological factors, elements of the child's environment that may be exacerbating a primary cause, be secondary to it, or be maintaining it. The case history findings also provide data for evaluating prognosis and the variables and constraints in progress that intervention will have to be adjusted to. This data may assume added significance in examining children where reliable language and intellectual measures are absent. Standard areas of enquiry in the diagnostic interview include the medical history, motor and sensory milestones and social development. Clinicians have routine questions and expected answers on which judgements of normal/ non-normal development are based. To gain a reliable picture of people from different cultural traditions it is necessary to be aware of normal variations in the patterns of upbringing, socialisation and attitudes to disorders which might otherwise lead the interviewer to erroneous conclusions. It is impossible to cover here all the beliefs of all communities, and all intracommunal variations. Suffice it to say that it is false to expect cultural homogeneity in ethnic minority groups any more than one would across dominant culture subgroups, and so clinicians' and educationalists' aims should be to acquaint themselves with local beliefs and practices.

A brief overview follows of the areas in which differences might be expected and the nature of some of those differences. As the experience of the author lies chiefly with Indian and West Indian children, more examples are taken from those communities, but this does not of course mean other cultures do not manifest variations.

Ethnic Minorities and Western Health

The first obstacle is actually encouraging ethnic minority members to utilise a health service created for and controlled by dominant culture interests. There are hurdles for any consumers at two levels – the institutional and the personal.

For immigrant families there will be considerable differences between the mechanics of operation of the health services in their country of origin and present abode. Henley (1979, 1980) describes how the British National Health Service (NHS) differs from health care in India. Indian consumers not used to the role of the general practitioner (GP), the need to make appointments, and system of GP referrals to hospital departments, with all its accompanying bureaucracy, tend to go directly to hospital outpatients' departments where according to their Indian experience they would expect to be seen. Mares (1981) discusses the contrasts between the former North and South Vietnam health services and the problems faced by Vietnamese in encountering the NHS.

Having ascertained that in Britain one goes initially to a GP's house practice or local health centre, and having found out how one actually receives an interview there, both no mean feat, there still remain problems of knowing who to go to, the range of services offered and under what circumstances one attends. Immigrants, even less than locally-born people, are unlikely to appreciate the relative roles of the GP, health visitor, school medical officer, social worker, hearing therapist, speech pathologist and chemist. Also, if they have not experienced it in their country of origin, they are unlikely to appreciate the significance of attendance at antenatal clinics, for immunisations, developmental checks, and the fact that health personnel may come to them uninvited (at school, work and home) when they are feeling well. Such visits require careful planning and explanation to allay common fears that one is from the 'authorities' and has come to collect evidence that may result in the refusal of work or residence permits, or deportation. Problems associated with home visits are discussed further in Chapter 10.

For immigrants the idea may be alien that health care workers come to offer advice on subjects that to them are either the private business of the family or not perceived as 'health' matters, e.g. toilet training, choice of toys, feeding, preparation and storage of food or financial aid available. The importance of prophylaxis and the non-acute services available (including long-term remediation of physical, mental and other developmental or acquired handicaps) need to be explained also.

Language constitutes a major hurdle, both in struggling to contact the right agency within a strange system and in actually discussing matters when the agency is reached. D. Smith (1977) claimed that in Britain as many as 77 per cent of Pakistani and Bangladeshi women spoke little or no English, while the figure for Indian women was 60 per cent and 41 per cent for African Asians. Nowotny (1976) found language a significant barrier in getting Asian women to use the NHS effectively. Even those willing to attend may be unable to because clinic times clash with when their interpreter husband or brother is working.

Language and cultural conceptual differences contribute to difficulties of communication at the personal level. Once a person has reached the agency they wish to contact, they still have to explain why they are there and comprehend in return the health worker's reply. Attitudes to what constitutes a problem warranting health service referral, describing that problem and ideas concerning its aetiology and satisfactory treatment all show cross-cultural variation. Views on health, illness and recovery may be still heavily influenced by religious and folk beliefs on the geography and functioning of the body. Belief in the power of evil spirits is still widespread (see Mares, 1981, and Okunade, 1981) despite considerable contact with Western medical methods. Hoyle (1981) reports the instance of an Asian mother of a hearing-impaired child believing the child's deafness resulted from her having been rude to a deaf boy when she was young. A degree of fatalism also can be found. If a person feels a disability has been sent by a deity, or that it is a stroke of bad luck, they may not see it as a condition that can be ameliorated.

The role of the four humours is still believed in, their link with the four elements, wind, earth, fire and air, and in turn their properties of wet, dry, hot and cold. Illnesses, medicines and food may be described in these terms. Frequently families may incur great debts to consult ethnic healers who know how to redress the balance of humours or how to counteract curses and evil spirits. Okunade (1981) has analysed the beliefs regarding possibilities, cause and treatment of handicap in Nigerian traditional, semi-traditional and Westernised settings. Ross (1980) discusses the importance of traditional healers, *hakims* and *vaids*, in the Asian community. West Indians may visit the *obeah* man (or woman), Muslims a *mowvli*. Chinese may rely on acupuncturists and bone-setters. Gil (1981) discusses the use of *espiritismo* in Puerto Rican mothers' attitudes towards their own and children's mental health problems. Treatment in these cases might consist of various herbal preparations, the laying on of hands, manipulation of body parts or observing certain rituals. These people may be attended, in addition to a Western health centre, or instead of, especially if a person feels their problem has not been properly understood or treated.

A common complaint from health care workers is that ethnic minorities plague surgeries with trivial ailments and yet neglect serious conditions. This stems partly from an ignorance of the terms of reference of different agencies, partly from beliefs about the capabilities of Western medicine, and partly from the implications of illnesses in different cultures. Coming from a background where contracting a chill might be fatal, where abdominal pain might be associated with diseases much more serious than a minor gastric upset, and a cough might be taken as a sure sign of tuberculosis, it is not surprising that these symptoms should cause such alarm.

Further, variation occurs in how pain or discomfort should be shown. On a world scale the English stiff upper lip is an isolated phenomenon and other cultures would feel they would not be taken seriously or that they were only 'putting it on' unless they gave full verbal and physical expression to their illness. Many Western clinicians might interpret these symptoms as having a psychosomatic basis on account of the apparent 'hysteria'. This conclusion may be reinforced by descriptions of a sore head as, pointing to the pelvic region, 'starting here and coming up'. The location and description of disorders has considerable cross-cultural variation and the clinician would benefit from awareness of the beliefs of particular communities with which they might be working.

In contrast to apparent over-concern for certain conditions, others, particularly if there is no associated (painful) physical sign, may not be recognised, or may be concealed because of the stigma attached to it. Persons suffering physical and mental handicap, mental illness, asthma, TB, leprosy and deafness, even though the family might give them every support possible, may be kept hidden (literally and in conversation) because of the loss of prestige that would affect the whole family if the facts were known. Hence there may be potent community pressures against accepting a diagnosis of abnormal development, and in case history interviews families may be reluctant to admit the presence of handicaps in other relatives.

Certain expectations exist regarding the questions that will be asked concerning disorders and the intervention that is deemed appropriate. From the herbal and faith healing tradition medicinal preparations, physical contact and discussion are expected, and the same is sought from Western services. To be told to come back in a week or six months, or to be handed a prescription without a full explanation, is taken as an uncaring manner or even a sign of incompetence, especially if the client felt that questions asked were remote from the cause and course of the complaint as they see it. Referrals on to audiologists, speech pathologists or whatever may seem puzzling to people accustomed to receiving a comprehensive service from one person, and clients may arrive in a paediatric assessment centre with little or distorted views on why they are there. It is in this atmosphere that the *hakims* and *obeah* healers flourish, with their careful attention to all the person's ills, a familiarity with their perceptions of disorders, and, with their physical and explanatory contact, fulfilling their expectations of treatment.

The family, then, that arrives with their child(ren) for a developmental assessment has already surmounted numerous bureaucratic and cultural communication hurdles. There may be a dissatisfaction with how they have been handled to date, and confused impressions of why they are there and what will be done. It is in this context that the case history is taken. Again, it is impossible to document here all the normal different patterns of socialisation interviewers should be alert to, nor does space permit coverage of all the childhood illnesses children from other countries might have been exposed to. It is only possible to offer some examples of the types of differences.

Case History Taking

To avoid unnecessary friction it is helpful to know what names to address persons by – which are their personal names, which their family names, which their religious or caste names and which order these are given in. Some of a person's names may only be used by certain family members, while there might be taboos against writing or speaking names of religious significance. All family members do not necessarily share common surnames, and titles marking female and male are common.

It is also prudent to establish the family member to whom questions should be addressed and who is responsible for decision-making in the family. Explanations and courses of action are more likely to be followed if they have been made through the correct channels.

In taking personal data, awareness is also drawn to age assignment in many cultures, whereby a child is labelled one year old when born, two after one year and so on. Avoiding errors here can save serious misreadings on norm scales. Without the western preoccupation with time and dates and the obsession that baby is doing all the right things at the right time, many other cultures will have little concern for the dates of particular milestones and illnesses, and parental reports may be even more unreliable than usual for this reason.

Enquiries of childhood illnesses must be made in the light of comments above regarding perceptions of pain, disease and attitudes thereto. Exposure of immigrant children in their native country to diseases that may affect development not generally found amongst North American or North European children must be borne in mind. Thalassaemia and sickle cell anaemia are not uncommon amongst children from the Mediterranean, Caribbean, Africa and Asia, with its accompanying pain and lethargy; neither is rickets and its effect on bone growth and walking. A higher incidence of lead poisoning and its side effects on development has been mentioned by Lobo (1978) and Edgerton (1979). This may be from cooking utensils with a high lead content, but also from the lead-based medicinal and cosmetic *surma* (see also, Ross, 1980) which is widely applied to Asian children. The consequences of maternal and infant malnutrition at critical stages in development should not be forgotten (cf. Edgerton, 1979, and Glaser, 1982).

There are, apart from the availability of food, cultural observances and traditional diet, other variations in feeding. Infants may be breast-fed for up to a year, not necessarily always by their own mother. When ill the child may be fed only certain foods (see the notions of 'hot' and 'cold' above) and particular dietary regimes are seen as inducing or retarding favourable development. Birth weights and growth norm charts have been devised essentially on white Europeans. Lobo (1978) mentions the tendency for Asian babies to have lower average birth weight without being 'at risk', while West Indian babies are similar to British norms.

West Indian similarities in weight contrast with their precociousness in reaching motor milestones, with a reported (Lobo, 1978, p. 17) average advantage according to British scales of three months. In communities where children are carried around on adults' backs well into childhood, the willingness and refined skills of walking may be delayed, though of course the underlying capacity should become apparent on testing.

The centrality of the mother-child relationship is another white middle-class obsession. There exist cross-cultural differences without accompanying deviancy in child development. There may be different main caretakers as well as variation in the child-rearing practices and expectations. One might contrast the position of the West Indian with the Indian child. The former, while their mother works, may be brought up by a grandmother, maternal aunt, older sister or cousin, if their services are available, otherwise be sent to a child-minder. A fixed father figure is not present in the traditional West Indian family unit, and the persons who might fill this role would tend to change more or less often. In effect they are single-parent families, but the same stigma is not attached to them as in white suburbia. This does not mean that the middle-class controlled British social services do not discriminate against what they see as an anomaly. In contrast, the Indian child will be cared for by his mother within the extended family, where this is intact, and will relate to a number of adults as main caregivers, though the eldest male will have ultimate authority. Where the trend has been towards a more nuclear family Anglo/British patterns may predominate, or (unregistered) child-minders are resorted to.

The treatment of the child may also vary. The white middle-class emphasis on individual action, initiative, competitiveness and material gain with respect for, but not dependence on, the parents is stressed elsewhere. Indian and Mediterranean (Triseliotis, 1976) children, on the other hand, may be kept highly dependent on their parents until school entry, to the extent that all their requirements will be fulfilled without them needing to 'earn' them. On entry to school, however, they may be expected to take on responsibility for household chores, the upbringing of younger siblings and participation in any family businesses. Again, this contrasts to communities where children must acquire early self-dependence.

Many more dimensions of variation can be found which can only be mentioned here – discipline and punishment (physical, ridicule, verbal) in the family and expected treatment of the child at school (Triseliotis, 1976, Noble and Ryan, 1976), the emotional implications of immigration and attendant family separation, culture shock and opposing sets of (age- and community-related) values (C. Ballard, 1979); and the role of language (as regulator of behaviour, in play, seen but not heard syndrome) within the family and wider group, are all recognised variables.

Some clinicians follow, if not explicitly, then at least implicitly, in their assessment, developmental charts, such as Gunzburg (1975), Sheridan (1975), Jeffree and McConkey (1976). Employed properly these are useful tools, but just as with standardised tests extreme caution must be exercised in applying them in a cross-cultural milieu.

The foregoing has highlighted some of the more obvious areas for misinterpretation. It is up to clinicians to enlighten themselves on other people's conceptions and their own misconceptions, and at the same time to work to create a health service which provides for all and not just one cultural elite.

10 MANAGEMENT OF COMMUNICATION PROBLEMS IN BILINGUAL CHILDREN

Niklas Miller and Sam Abudarham

What is the Problem?

The question is better phrased: what are the problems? Essentially they divide into three – the child's, the therapist's and the community's. The problems centred on the child include his primary handicapping condition – mental retardation, specific learning disorder, hearing impairment, etc. – and their associated difficulties. These may be classified as medical, social, emotional, motor and cognitive, including language. The central concern of this book has been defining a language handicap in a bilingual setting, and this chapter on management is directed chiefly at this, though naturally considering it in its social-emotional context.

The problems centred on the therapist/teacher, as outlined in the preface, derive from attempts to assess a bilingual's potential with monolingual tools; and having found a solution to that, how one is to apply remediation with monolingual methods. The bilingual setting throws up a host of questions that Western professional training has not provided answers for: what language(s) is to be used in therapy; what form does therapy need to take; what methods can one employ to carry out therapy in a language one has no knowledge of; how and when does therapy in two languages start; can one rely on the same principles and practices of intervention familiar from monolingual settings; how is one to work with an ethnic minority family who may speak no English? Difficulties here may lead to a serious gap if the therapist/teacher cannot count on the understanding and cooperation from home which would normally be necessary. Understanding the implications of language choice, handicap and differences in other-culture expectations and wishes represents a further novel area of consideration for most workers. The problems faced by the other-culture family that the remediator will need to be aware of cannot be underestimated.

Most of these difficulties derive from the third category, the community-centred problems. The above only become problem issues in a society that is run by and for monolinguals and that makes no provision for the diversity within its bounds. If there were proper facilities for bilingual education and equal access to rights and institutions irrespective of language background the problem of the bilingual child could be treated to all intents and purposes like the monolingual child. As it is, provisions are scarce, and thus semilingualism (q.v.), limited English proficiency and remediators' monolingual materials become problems, and in addition to their primary handicapping condition, society imposes further hindrances on the bilingual child. In its ignorance, Western scholarship and society has laid the fault of many of the consequences of its own narrow functioning at the door of the bilingual-bicultural and it is they who are seen as needing adjustment, not society as a whole. In this way English as a second language becomes a 'problem' often leading to erroneous placement in special schools; other-culture behaviour is seen as maladaptive and people are labelled as behavioural or psychiatric problems. Haberland and Skutnabb-Kangas (1979), Skutnabb-Kangas (1981), Cheng *et al.* (1979) and J. Edwards (1981) have addressed issues in community-centred problems and their negative side-effects for the individual.

The following guidelines for management of communication problems in the bilingual child are made in the context of the imperfect, discriminatory situation as it at present stands. It is acknowledged that a genuine solution, rather than stop-gap measures, will only be forthcoming following wider societal change. It is not within the scope of this chapter to say how this should be brought about, but that is not to discourage those who would struggle to hasten the arrival of that day.

Principles of Management

This chapter concerns only the management of speech and language problems. It does not intend to cover disorders of voice and fluency. Differences and difficulties do exist between cultures regarding what is considered as an acceptable degree of dysfluency or what is to be taken as a voice disorder. However, a discussion of these fields would be out of place in this volume which has concentrated on speech and language.

Sound management presupposes that a correct differential diagnosis has been made. The difficulties in arriving at a differential diagnosis with regard to whether the child has a (first) language learning problem or a second language learning problem, have already been highlighted and discussed in other publications (Abudarham, 1980a, 1980b and 1982; and Gavillán, this volume). Whereas no objective, valid and reliable test instrument is available as yet, circumstantial evidence from observations and case history data can often point to one particular diagnosis. Clearly a false diagnosis could lead to waste of valuable time and cause undue frustration to both client and therapist and not least to the client's family. Assessment must have ascertained a reliable estimate of the child's stage of development, his needs, his strengths and weaknesses and the possible cause(s) of his language delay. Management will be different for the child with limited proficiency due to hearing loss or mental handicap and those limited only because of their unsuitable exposure to a variety of languages.

No management plans can be formulated in ignorance of the individual's needs. It is easy to suggest activities one can do 'as a general rule' without paying due heed to the exact nature of the child's problems and factors such as those militating against his linguistic progress or those which would enhance such development. One therefore needs to know as many aspects as possible of this 'syndrome' called 'bilingualism' or 'dual language' (Abudarham, 1980a, b). Factors such as how long the child has been in this country, how long he has been exposed to the English language, the exact nature of his linguistic background, i.e. what language, or languages, are spoken at home; parental attitudes to him as a child, his problems and the learning and/or speaking of English at home, will all determine the way he can be helped. One cannot, of course, forget that this is a 'child' with a problem and not a 'problem' in a child. Whatever considerations are made in developing management plans for a monoglot have still to be made for a child with dual languages. This means that investigations made through the medium of interviews and case history taking apply to both the dual language child and the monoglot. Questions related to birth circumstances, developmental milestones, hereditary factors, etc. are just as relevant as might be psychometric, paediatric and other investigations by other agencies. It would be presumptuous of anyone to attempt to lay down hard and fast rules about the exact form that therapy should take. It would also be misleading, for just as this could not be done for any pathological condition in a group of monoglots, it is not feasible for a bilingual child. However, one can discuss therapeutic principles.

The fact that there are certain principles that can be applied to the communication-disordered population at large cannot be denied. There is no reason why the same should not be true for bilingual patients. After all, once a (first) language problem is diagnosed, at this point the bilingual patient is in the same category as the monoglot patient – both share a difficulty in learning language. In the case of the (potential) bilingual child, however, his linguistic environment is different at home to the one outside. He, therefore, not only has difficulty in learning language but he also has to contend with two different linguistic codes. Whereas there will be common rules in both codes, there will almost certainly be many more which are different or, worse still, in opposition.

One question invariably raised is what language(s) therapy should be conducted in. There is no hard and fast rule that can be applied in answer to this, and every case must be evaluated on an individual basis. Some concrete examples may serve to illustrate issues and influences that may be involved.

Gopal was a three-year-old Punjabi child with very little comprehension and a reported twelve words in Punjabi. He had a mild spastic diplegia and had suffered from hypoglycaemia. Members of the team had opposing views about the best way to proceed. The educational psychologist and teacher recommended that Gopal be taught English since that was the teaching medium at school. The speech therapist counselled that it was more important to encourage the mother-child relationship via play, and of course in Punjabi, since the mother could not speak much English and was not likely to want to learn English. At first sight this seemed a rational approach. However, further discussion revealed that the child was unlikely to be able to learn more than a few words a month. The suggestion was then made that his mother be approached and encouraged to learn those words in English that were going to be taught in school so that she could reinforce them when appropriate. She could also be taught key words to do with the child's immediate environment and needs. It seemed reasonable to expect that mother could learn English faster than Gopal could learn Punjabi or English. Teaching the child words in two languages seemed uneconomical since it was very likely that some of the words learned in the two languages would refer to one object or concept. Very often, one meets with opposition to this type of advice from parents of some ethnic groups. These parents see part of the role of the educationalist as teaching English to their children whereas they see themselves as responsible for teaching their children their own language. They therefore resent any suggestion that they should speak to their children in a second language and refuse to do so. One mother who could not speak English once argued that there was little use in speaking to her child if he could not understand her. One must respect the strength and logic of such a view.

Simon was referred by his parents at the age of three. His father talked to him in Yiddish, his mother in English and the child was also being taught to read and pray in Hebrew. In normal circumstances, coping with three languages is a feasibility. Jewish children living in bilingual communities usually have no difficulty in doing this, and indeed there are other communities, such as in parts of Switzerland or Kenya, where children are also exposed to three languages. However, the problem arises when the child is finding it difficult to learn even one language. This is even more significant with children with severe language-learning problems. The aim should be to maximise the number of referrents to which the child can attach a verbal label. An individual has a finite language-learning potential. This potential usually exceeds his communicative needs. But this is often not the case with children with language-learning problems. It therefore seems sensible not to exhaust a possibly severely reduced potential by teaching the child two lexical items (i.e. one in each language) for each referrent. Arguably, if two languages were used one could find that out of a total vocabulary repertoire of say fifty words, eighteen in L1 and eighteen in L2 could be synonymous, so that the 'naming' power of such a vocabulary might only cover thirty-two referrents. This would not seem to be the best way of capitalising on the available potential. Simon's parents, therefore, were urged to speak to him in one language alone. They were told that it was up to them what language they chose to speak to their child in, but that the speech therapist could help them reach that decision if they so wished. After discussion, Simon's father reluctantly agreed to concentrate on English. Simon received speech therapy and after a year reached a language level within normal limits for his age. When the speech therapist was satisfied that Simon had consolidated this level, his parents were then advised that he could probably cope with more intensive exposure to other languages. This advice has been given several times and has proved successful.

Leila was a four-year old Down's syndrome child born in Britain, who for the first eighteen months of her life had been exposed at home to English. This was from her English father, her mother who was bilingual in English and Arabic and her brother who was two years older. At eighteen months she had been sent to her mother's country of origin to be brought up by her grandmother until her mother's intended return. However, on account of the war situation in that country, she returned at age three and a half to the UK with her aunt. During her stay she had been exposed only to Arabic. In the interim her mother had separated from her husband, and so on her return Leila could still have been addressed only in Arabic, except for two factors.

The first was that her brother had entered an English medium school and forgotten most of his Arabic. His mother had not wanted him to be disadvantaged on starting school and so had spoken to him solely in English during the past year or so. The second factor was that Leila was attending an English language preschool group for mentally handicapped children. The family fully intended leaving Britain after the mother had completed her studies in one or two year's time.

The dilemma was that by not being taught English Leila was being excluded from the developmentally facilitating environment of the playgroup. Balanced against this was the fact that the other children in the group had three and a half years start over her in English, however quickly she might learn (she was only mildly retarded according to non-verbal observations and measures). This was a factor that therapy would simply have had to overcome had her residence in Britain been permanent. The fact, though, that she would eventually have to function in an Arabic-speaking community made it seem pointless to expose her to yet another language switch, a move that would be reversed yet again when she left the country. The compromise reached was that her aunt (who could understand English) should attend the playgroup with her. The playgroup leader undertook to learn some of Leila's active Arabic vocabulary, which at that stage was not very extensive, and the mother and aunt were to reintroduce the brother to Arabic. This would have the dual advantage of permitting verbal interaction between the siblings at home and of preparing the brother for the move back to the Arabic setting. The speech therapist was to train the aunt in therapeutic techniques and content, which she then, under the therapist's supervision, applied in Arabic.

If none of these cases seems typical this only serves to emphasise the diversity of situations likely to be encountered and the difficulty in dictating global non-specific solutions. Bearing in mind the threshold and developmental interdependence hypotheses (q.v.) it would seem that concentrating on one language at a time is advisable with children with limited language proficiency. The problem is arriving at a decision on what language and when to introduce a second language. These decisions have to be met with a consideration of all the sociocultural aspects that are going to impinge on the child's linguistic needs, and how far therapeutic possibilities and overall development are going to render hopes realistic. Thus as well as the child's language strengths and weaknesses, and communicative needs, remediators may also need to take into account the wishes of individual families. Their wishes must be stressed, since the language used at home is a choice fraught with emotive cultural and social connotations. If a choice, for whatever reasons, has to be made contrary to the wishes of the family, they must be reassured that this is only a means to an end, permitting a later choice to be made to their favour, rather than the decision representing an immutable end in itself. It is not the task of therapists to alter religious or cultural values, but it is their task, as exhaustively and as sympathetically as possible, to explain and discuss with families the full range of possibilities and the long- and short-term implications of any decisions.

The initial aim in remediation should be to develop communicative proficiency in keeping with mental age in at least one language. A child is more likely to be successful at acquiring a second language if development in the first has been maximal. Further, the developmental interaction between language and cognition is only likely to be fully realised if progress in language is fully exploited. Dissipating the potential of a child with limited proficiency by exposing him to conflicting codes would in general not seem the most efficient teaching strategy. If a second language is eventually introduced it should be kept as a cardinal point that ongoing progress in the first language must not be neglected if a state of semilingualism is to be avoided. On occasions, for whatever reason, two languages may have to be learned simultaneously. The aim in such instances would be to ensure that there existed maximum predictability for the child regarding who uses what language and where the language is used.

It is clear that no one profession on its own can tackle the linguistic problem. To some extent, and if we are to believe in the potency of a team approach, this is true about the monoglot patient. Evidently, it is truer of the bilingual child, except that the team is more likely to be joined by, possibly, a community worker, a teacher of English as a second language and an interpreter. The need for parental cooperation becomes more poignant than in the case of the monoglot child. It is our contention that the roles of the different agencies need not vary from those adopted for the monolingual child, although the position of the speech pathologist/therapist with expertise in language development may acquire extra importance. This may not only be in the more complex situation presented by bilingualism, but also as a counsellor and guide to other workers involved. The school teacher likewise has added responsibility, not only in the increased vigilance in home-school-clinic liaison, but also because he or she may have to cope with the results of any errors made at the diagnostic stage. He or she may also be the professional person who is most likely to have the best opportunity to recommend alternative schooling if a child has been misplaced. The greatest dilemma in this area can be found in special schools which often become dumping grounds for children who 'normal' schools cannot or do not wish to cope with.

The position of the teacher of English as a second language (ESL) is worth noting in this context. In one's experience they are the ones most susceptible to being landed with problems. One of the reasons for this is that authorities often appoint these teachers to special schools and teachers there are not aware of the inadequacy of using ESL techniques with children with (first) language learning problems and instinctively turn to teachers of ESL when they have bilingual children in their classes. Also, possibly, the ESL training schools do not seem to alert teachers to the fact that they are not trained to cope with first-language learning problems and other pathological conditions, e.g. mental retardation, cerebral palsy, etc. Furthermore, the teacher of ESL is not trained to recognise a first-language learning problem, as distinct to a second-language learning problem. Arriving at the differential diagnosis is difficult enough for speech therapists (Abudarham, 1980a, b, 1982). Ideally, all cases of suspected first-language problems met by the teacher of ESL should be referred for assessment by the speech therapist who can make in-depth investigations which will provide a differential diagnosis. Sometimes, a child's medical condition or severe cognitive problems may suggest that he is likely to have a first-language learning problem. Total absence or severe paucity of any language at all could suggest the same.

The rule of thumb should be that if a second-language learning problem is indicated, the teacher of English as a second language should intervene. However, if there is evidence of a (first) language learning problem, the speech therapist should be the primary remediator. A note of caution is appropriate at this point. Sometimes children are referred with no knowledge of English and it soon becomes clear that they have only a very primitive first language, or none at all. These cases are often seen in the reception and nursery classes in special schools. The role of the teacher of English as a second language, in such cases, must be minimal if at all. There is little point in many of these cases in employing ESL teaching techniques when the child has not got even one language.

Reasons for this are numerous. Many techniques used in teaching ESL are often counterproductive when used with some children suffering from language problems, especially those with language disorders. We have seen the results of this when the problems peculiar to such conditions are not and cannot be fully understood by the ESL teacher. For example, a common teaching strategy in ESL is not to teach words in isolation but within a 'sentence' framework. This is right and proper when teaching children who can apply grammatical rules given different linguistic contexts. However, some educationally subnormal children cannot do this and learn the rule parrot-fashion. When shown a series of pictures and asked what they were, an Asian child with a language disorder responded using the framework 'this is a . . .'. The child used this framework regardless of whether the picture was of an object whose name started with a vowel or whether there was more than one object, thus 'this is a apple' and 'this is a shoes' were examples of such replies. This child was nine years old.

ESL teachers may be valuable team members if parents need to be taught a second language parallel to their child's learning. After proficiency has been established in a first language and the time comes to introduce a second language, ESL teachers may play an important part. Tough (1977) discusses the principles and practices to be considered in when and how to introduce a second language to young normal children, principles which it would be advisable for clinicians to know in forming effective working partnerships with ESL teachers. Tosi (this volume) covers the scope of bilingual education and second-language programmes.

The assessment and teaching of hearing-impaired and deaf children poses special difficulties. Conducting pure-tone audiometry, stapedial reflex-testing and similar objective measures should be possible with the aid of an efficient interpreter. However, for various reasons it may be necessary to carry out speech audiometry or word discrimination testing. Using English language words will clearly produce unreliable indications of a child's potential, even though the same results might show the level at which they are likely to function in an English medium classroom. McLauchlin (1980) discusses the use of speech protocols with children of limited language ability amongst which he includes non-English-speaking persons. He deals briefly with the problems of the availability of foreign speech materials, how these are to be presented and what type of listener response is appropriate. Martin and Hart (1978) investigated and confirmed the feasibility of a prerecorded Spanish speech threshold procedure, using a picture pointing format that could be administered by non-Spanish-speaking clinicians. Their test used Texas Spanish, so would not be generally acceptable for all Spanish-speakers. However, they concluded that the procedure employed in developing the test should be appropriate in devising speech audiometric assessments in other regional dialects and languages.

In the education of the hearing-impaired bilingual child, the language 'problems', as with hearing children, centre around the choice of what language(s) to choose and when. The educational stages and objectives after these decisions have been made should not need to differ radically from those with monoglots. The additional complications encountered stem from the different sociocultural context to which decisions have to be suited. Luetke (1976), in her survey of Mexican-American parents of hearing-impaired children, found a big gap between the services imposed by a monolingual-oriented education system and the desires of the bilingual families. She also found a serious shortage of literature which might offer assistance to remediation in the hearing field, a state of affairs which has been only slightly ameliorated in the interim. Hoyle (1980) from her experience also points to the sociocultural factors that add to the difficulties faced by children from non-English-speaking homes, many of them deriving from parents' poor knowledge of the causes of hearing loss and the function of teachers of the deaf and their aims and methods. Hearing-impaired children with their greater reliance on non-verbal signs are also more susceptible to cross-cultural differences in facial expression, use of gesture and tone of voice.

Lerman (1980) describes one project designed to train educators in the special needs of Hispanic hearing-impaired children. Like Hoyle, he underlined the fact that attempts to offer improved services often founder on the poor adaptability of present educational provisions and reluctance of state departments to make available adequate support. He also approached the subject of which language to choose in instruction, suggesting that children below four years should be taught in their home language, thereby fostering a close relationship to the family, giving the developmental advantages that this can offer. Children with losses below seventy decibels could be considered dominant in their home language and the principles of bilingual education could be applied. Lerman would support offering Spanish language systems to adolescents where previous years of English instruction have not been beneficial. Oxman (1975) details a reception programme for hearing-impaired children and though her results proved negative, at least they provide lessons for others' endeavours.

Remediation Methods and Materials

It is not within the scope of this chapter to discuss remedial speech therapy techniques in detail. There are other worthy textbooks which achieve this end very competently. Our view has been that the core content of remediation for 'bilinguals' does not need to differ from that utilised with the monolingual child. They both have the same problem – a first-language learning difficulty – and the ultimate goal with both is the same – communicative competence and independence. The differences lie in the concomitant factors that need to be considered in planning and executing intervention. Again this is nothing new, since remediators are obliged with any child to take into consideration the wider implications of a person's history and background when devising programmes. The more problematical areas concern arriving at an accurate assessment and actually applying remedial measures. These matters have been the subject of this whole book. Some brief mention might be made of areas of concern required with bilingual children not commonly encountered amongst monoglots.

The arguments between creative learning 'errors' and other-language interference were outlined in Chapter 4. Whichever side one supports on that issue, there will be some examples of interlanguage interference not acceptable to the linguistic community, that may need remediation. In the child's phonological development there may be well-established patterns related to L1 that make the production of new articulatory placements difficult to achieve. Vowel distortion particularly can lead to impairment of intelligibility, not only from contrasting vowel systems, but also the effect that vowel length might have on consonant perception and production. Different systems of contrast may lead to confusions between fortis-lenis or aspirated-non-aspirated consonants. Speakers of Hindi, Gujarati and Urdu often produce English initial voiceless aspirated consonants as unaspirated, which are perceived by native English-speakers as voiced consonants. Thus *pea* might be taken as *bee*, *cards* as *guards* and so on. Stress, pitch, rhythm and intonation may also require therapy. Stress variations can bring about misunderstandings. Thus pairs such as home-sick v. home sick, toy-shop v. toy shop are susceptible to misinterpretation and mispronunciation, apart from the wider, less local effects altered stress timing might have on intelligibility for the listener. The affective consequences of altered prosodic features were mentioned in Chapters 3 and 4. Intonation plays an important part in pre-spoken language development and early one- and two-word phrase production. Contrasting models, both from the foreign languages and the Indian-English or Latino-English of their peers and family in comparison with standard British or American English, could conceivably lead to false comprehension by the child of intonational cues, as well as false or inconsistent production on their part.

It would be our recommendation that one treats only those aspects of other-language influence that impair intelligibility. It should also go without saying that one does not attempt to alter features of locally current norms any more than one would attempt to treat any other local accent of English. For instance, one feature of what is loosely termed 'Indian English' is the tendency to realise alveolar consonants with a degree of retroflexion. The remediators should be aware of group characteristics like these and in their assessment exclude them from any decisions concerning the presence of a disorder.

In syntax, interference in word order may need therapy. This may include the order of clause-level constitutents – subject, verb, object – and dependent clauses; or phrase level constitutents – pre- and post-positions, adjectival placements, realisation of determiners, as well as number and tense marking. If a second language is introduced, either as a second language, or with the intention of it eventually becoming the child's L1, it is prudent to commence learning with those elements of language over which the child already has command and that have identical or near identical structural characteristics in both L1 and L2.

The same holds for the introduction of lexical items. One should introduce first labels for items with which the child is familiar and not those where exist cross-cultural differences in either occurrence or organisation. Common examples of the latter include colour terms, kinship taxonomies and verbs of motion – come, go, bring, take, walk, run, ride, etc. – which might follow conventions of usage at variance between L1 and L2 (cf. also pages 74-5).

Very little has been written on remedial programmes for 'bilingual' language-disordered children. Most literature is written either under the influence of ESL, ignoring the issues of establishing a first language in disordered children, or it explicitly or implicitly furthers the view that all children *must* acquire English, irrespective of their background. Deignan and Ryan (1979) have compiled an annotated list of materials for the bilingual special education needs of Spanish-dominant children. They divide their bibliography into different skills areas, including auditory perceptual and language development. Bergin (1980) in her review of materials mentions the dearth of specifically designed bilingual-bicultural software for the limited proficient child, though she does identify some programmes and publications which go some way towards being suitable. To date, it remains largely up to individuals to adapt existing resources or create their own material for cross-cultural use. Ideally, any training of personnel in this field should include instruction in points of consideration in effecting this.

As well as reflecting the child's different cultural experience, materials might be introduced in a manner familiar to the child's background. An interesting move in this direction was tried by Harris (1978), who successfully adapted traditional aboriginal education methods (e.g. personal trial and error and observation and imitation versus conscious verbal instruction) practised within the tribe for use in mainstream Australian schools which the students had to attend. Other ways of capitalising on strategies familiar to children might be to use their own ethnic stories and story-telling techniques, as represented in the Language Support Services (1982) handbook; or build on their familiar verbal play, such as the verbal duelling of West Indians. Multilingual work displays and their use have been mentioned by V. Edwards (1981). Fair Play for Children (1982) introduces many games played by Asian and Caribbean children that could be gainfully adapted to therapeutic ends.

Home Visits

Much of the success of intervention will depend on establishing positive links with the child's home background. Workers need to be prepared for the altered conditions encountered in gaining such links. The different conceptions of illness, its cause and course, have already been mentioned elsewhere (p. 172), as have hurdles in using the health service and understanding the role of remediators. In addition to cultural differences arising out of these areas, home visiting presents its own points of contrast.

The following remarks apply mainly to work with people from an Indian subcontinent background, as this is the area most within the experience of the authors. For other immigrant or indigenous groups (e.g. in Wales, Ireland and Canada) other necessary adjustments and considerations must be established.

Arriving at a house unannounced is not a good start. If the person who normally negotiates in English with visitors and outside agencies, and the family decision-makers are not there, other members of the household (especially female members to male callers) may not answer the door. An introductory communication explaining the purpose of the visit is highly recommended. The idea of the 'caring' professions may be alien to people who have relied on the corporate expertise of the extended family in matters pertaining to child-rearing, illness and family 'problems'. There may be a feeling initially that this is an interfering outsider prying into private affairs. The attitude may be that teachers/therapists have their role (taken that this is recognised, an assumption that cannot be made) and parents' theirs, and they have their locations in which they exercise their respective authority. The desire to visit a home to discuss teaching matters may seem at least strange, and at most an admission of incompetence on the part of the remediator. Hence the importance of setting out beforehand the precise role of the visitor, the function of the visit and the mutual responsibilities and expectations for the parties.

Letters should be addressed to the head of the household, even if it was the mother and child seen alone in clinic. It is also the elders of the family who should be greeted on first entering a house. It is they who may have the ultimate word in decisions on therapy, school placement or whatever, and even if they cannot speak English their superior position should be acknowledged. Later on it may be expected that questions be directed through one responsible member of the family, even if the issues concern other members. Women might not speak in the presence of husbands, brothers or fathers. Certain matters may be taboo or require careful introduction. Other subjects must be discussed with the whole family, even when the matter involves only one individual. In extended family units children are seen as the responsibility of the whole family, not just the immediate parents. The mother's mother-in-law may have as much say in the child as the mother herself, and she is responsible for her daughter-in-law's behaviour. It is not usually proper for a male visitor to interview a female person alone. Other cultural etiquette must be observed. It is well to be acquainted with what counts as an offering of hospitality, obligatory topics of conversation prior to the main business of a visit, and the expectations of the family regarding the visitor as well as vice versa. In Western health services case history taking, interviewing and counselling are accepted as one-sided affairs – the health worker asks or instructs, the client responds. The Western health worker may be unprepared for personal questions and demands directed in turn at him, yet this is something that may be encountered. He may also be expected to accept gifts and attend family functions. To decline may be taken as a sign of ingratitude. As well as awareness of what might be taken as intentional and unintentional impolite behaviour, the health worker should also monitor his own dress, nature of questioning and etiquette (who sits where, who talks to whom, etc.) to avoid causing offence. Such cautions as above are all advisable in establishing an atmosphere of trust in which therapy and cooperation might flourish.

The language barrier is a second major obstacle in carrying out effective intervention via the family. Besides an assessment of the child's language, an appraisal of the caretaker's skills in English is necessary, (1) for their understanding of questions and advice and directions given, and (2) for carrying out any therapy envisaged in English. Because a family can give biographical details and pass the time of day and even talk about matters of work in English, it does not follow that they will comprehend enquiries concerning medical and developmental history and correctly interpret instructions for them to carry out. This presents enough problems for monolingual parents, let alone for those operating in a foreign language, and coping with a situation which for them is an area of stress. Henley (1979, Chapter 12) offers guidelines both for optimising one's own use of English to ensure maximum intelligibility and for monitoring interviewee's comprehension of directions given. In aiming for highest efficiency in explanation and questioning she suggests, for instance, the use of a slowed, clearly spoken delivery (at a normal loudness and pitch but not word by word or pidgin English) not containing unnecessary jargon or unfamiliar words and idioms and avoiding complicated grammatical structures. The logical sequencing of questions and explanations should be thought out carefully beforehand to minimise confusion arising from constant switches from one unrelated point to another, and illustrative examples and accompanying visual and gestural material should be monitored to ensure that it actually supports the verbal message rather than runs counter to it.

To find out whether one has been correctly understood a useful tactic Henley offers is to develop a regular pattern of checking back, either by getting the person to demonstrate instructions or by questioning on individual points. Simply asking 'have you understood?' or accepting a smiling face and nods of the head as evidence for comprehension are not sufficient. One should be alert for clients who pretend they have followed things either because they are embarrassed or do not know how to request further explanation. Some clients may withhold some information or give up trying to elaborate on a matter important to them because they are unable to master the language necessary to convey it. On such occasions the health worker must give linguistic support, helping the person to explain themselves in easy stages that they can manage.

Interpreters

The services of an interpreter have often been recommended to help negotiate the language barrier. However, such a solution is far from the straightforward process it would seem, and wrongly employed can produce more negative effects than those experienced by the health worker struggling on alone – though Fitzgerald and McLachlan (1978, p. 34) with their examples of 'constipation' having been understood as diarrhoea and the fitting of a crown by a dental technician instead of the required filling by a dental surgeon, give ample warning of the dangers here. Rowell and Rack (1979) recommend that a clinical team should be not only multidisciplinary but also mutlilingual so that at least one member can *communicate* on behalf of the team, a task different from *interpreting* on their behalf. Short of this a *qualified* interpreter can be used. An interpreter plays an important part in the transcultural effectiveness of the team. Finding a suitable worker is the first step.

Unsuitable persons are considered to be those who have only a smattering or an inadequate command of either language involved. There is a vast difference between making oneself understood in limited contexts and translating specific, detailed, technical questions and instructions with fine gradations of meaning and relaying a reply accurately. But mastery of both languages is still not ideal – as Rowell and Rack (1979, p. 17) correctly maintain, 'To be fluently bilingual is not in itself a sufficient qualification for interpreting, anymore than the ability to write is in itself sufficient qualification for a secretary.' One needs a person who can transmit *exactly* what a person has requested, and likewise to reply. For this reason the interpreter requires not only a knowledge of the specialised vocabulary involved, but also an understanding of the aims of the interviewer, the willingness and ability to convey only what the questioner asks and only what the respondent replies. It is a frequent experience with poor interpreters to request them to elicit information which should require only a brief question, but the questioner is left standing for an unexpected time during a lengthy exchange before an answer is forthcoming. During an assessment session when an interpreter was being used, one of the authors explained to the interpreter in detail what was required. The latter was cautioned to ask only the question on the instruction sheet without adding or deleting any information. At one point the interpreter seemed to be taking an unexpectedly long time asking a question. The whole session had been videotaped and during discussion the interpreter admitted that he had asked the child to point at the 'bath'. The child did not respond correctly but he suspected the child knew what 'bath' meant. In trying to elicit a correct response the child had been asked to point 'at the thing next to the chair' (the child had previously responded correctly to 'chair').

The remediator should be alert for interpreters who make their own additions and false assumptions about questions, and filter replies, giving their own interpretation of a response rather than what the client really said. Make sure that the interpreter is not taking over control of a session and that the health worker is not losing rapport with the client. This can be a serious flaw during diagnostic and close counselling sessions.

A good interpreter should inform the questioner when they have difficulty translating and explain why. This may be due to the difficulty of translating some concepts, poor questioning on the health worker's side, a lack of understanding on the client's part, a shortcoming in the interpreters' skill or some extralinguistic factor. The latter two points require checking before commencing an interview. One should be assured beforehand that the interpreter is fluent in the client's language or dialect and that there exist no subcultural obstacles to smooth communication. For instance, members of different castes may on occasion be reluctant to speak to each other; the client/interpreter may be unwilling to break cultural conventions by discussing subjects which are mutually taboo or embarrassing. For this reason other family members do not provide the best interpreters.

Aside from their language and cultural knowledge, interpreters should ideally have personal skills that make them acceptable to clients, help put them at ease, do not offend or embarrass them, have a respect for confidentiality, maintain a neutral role, and be able to build a good working relationship with the health worker. Henley (1979) expands on many of the points raised regarding interpreters and covers others which space does not permit here.

Counselling and Parent Involvement

It has been taken as axiomatic in recent years that effective intervention with children and their problems must involve close cooperation with and of the parents. Where there exists a gulf between the family's understanding of a problem and a clinical team's perception of intervention, which is the rule rather than the exception in cross-cultural therapeutics, family counselling becomes not only a challenge but the *sine qua non* of good management. There are the barriers of language and cultural differences to break through. But there are also the understandable feelings of apprehensiveness, threat, guilt, shame and negativism to break through. It must be stressed that the health worker is not coming as a 'prying official' or as an agent of white health service imperialism, and that an awareness of cultural relativism must be adopted. Ethnic minorities have sets of values and traditions to observe which are as important to them as a white person's are to themselves. Any discussion, understanding and solutions must proceed from the client's own beliefs and values. Intervention that ignores, intentionally or not, these patterns is likely to be insulting, alien and unacceptable to the other community.

The ethnic minority's conceptions about the aetiology of a handicap in their child, however irrational they might seem, have to be taken as a starting point in the discussion of any feelings of recrimination or discord within the family. Attempting to impose willy-nilly Western thinking will meet with rejection. Non-appreciation of the cultural implications of having a handicapped child in the family will likewise lead to a breakdown of the therapeutic relationship. Unused to the idea that handicapped people have rights, potential and skills that can be developed, minority families who expect these handicapped people to be 'hidden' at home, may be reluctant or unclear about how to accept a remediator's plans for intervention. Differences in the role expectations and territory have already been mentioned above as factors which could result in non-acceptance of the 'intruding remediator'. The remoteness of the therapist's 'cure' from the way the cause and prognosis of the disorder is perceived by his family may be a further factor. Ideas of a child learning at its own rate through structured play and cognitive concept training may be as strange to parents from rural India or Mexico as the rote learning of facts and figures is to the Western urban dweller. Explaining to a family that their interaction with their child has to be modified and the environment restructured, apart from possibly not being understood, may be taken as direct or implied criticism of their ability to care for the child, and reinforce feelings that this is a prying official and not a caring therapist. Bedwetting, violence, emotional deprivation and other behaviour assumed to be maladaptive in the West will not necessarily be seen as 'problems', while other aspects may be.

The list could be endless, but the essential underlying message remains: one cannot assume that one's aims, however well meant, are going to be understood, accepted or appropriate. The culturally different client is not there to be adjusted to Western notions of what is right in therapy. Rather the client and his context form the starting point for the therapist to understand and adjust herself. From the start each move in assessment, diagnosis and therapy will have to be carefully evaluated for its suitability and effectiveness to the individual situation; its application will need thoughtful explanation and justification to the persons involved. Benjamin and Pratt (1975) cover the special needs of American Indians, Blacks, Chicanos and Mexican-Americans and training programmes for school counsellors with these ethnic groups. Christensen (1975) discusses some traits and values of Puerto Ricans and suggestions for counselling with them. Lobo (1978) and Saifullah-Khan (1979) deal with many of the background issues in working with Asian groups in Britain, while Lago and Ball (1983), as well as addressing the problem of helping in a multicultural context, offer a tentative checklist for counsellor training sessions.

Methods of involving parents have been attempted at various levels. These will be more or less useful according to the extent of information to be imparted and degree of involvement intended. Some health authorities have translated health education material on feeding, play and language development. This is all well and good, as long as one is sure parents are literate in their L1, that the remediator knows the content of the leaflets and is able to explain its relevance to the individual client. Simply handing over a booklet and telling someone to read it is no solution. A direct translation of Western material does not necessarily suit either, since it ignores the different background and expectations of other ethnic groups. Others have devised special materials, relying heavily on pictures, models and audiovisual techniques and have introduced them maybe as part of a community health education course run by health visitors, teachers or clinicians. An example is provided by the HELP Maternity Language Course (Lewycka, Mares and Whitaker, 1980) designed to instruct non-English-speaking mothers (-to-be) in the vocabulary and communication needed in ante- and post-natal clinics, as well as the British bureaucracy of childbirth.

The participation of parents in remediation has been achieved in other ways. Hahn and Dunston (1974) discuss their parent education approach; Quick (1976) describes the development of family learning centres for children needing language development; while Bergin (1980) and Wilson-Portuondo (1980) deal with the training of ethnic minority parents as paraprofessionals in teaching their own and other children from their ethnic group. In both health and education it has been found that commitment to and understanding of these systems is increased greatly when ethnic minority members are engaged in the design and delivery of the service as well as being its consumers. Further attempts at overcoming the difficulties of therapeutic application have made use of ESL classes being attended by parents. The language therapist has arranged with the ESL teacher to train the parents in areas of English which are going to be covered with their child.

Providing the Services Needed

Of course it does not have to be the parents who make the only effort. Efficiency of remedial services will be enhanced if personnel achieve fluency in minority languages, if staff can be recruited from the ethnic communities themselves and if proper provisions for bilingual or other-language education can be provided. These must be the ultimate aims of a service that wishes to succeed. In fact this is happening. In the interim the few persons who do offer these skills could be employed as peripatetic home tutors, for running parent education courses and as a central agent for advice, referrals and in-service training for non-bilingual/bicultural workers.

Pynn (1980) reports on a workshop held to identify the issues involved in the training and recruitment of staff for bilingual special education and the implementation of services. The workshop covered training courses that were in existence in the USA for workers entering the field of bilingual special education as well as defining areas in which trainees should become competent – namely, bicultural factors in learning; knowledge of the nature and needs of exceptional bilingual/bicultural children; speech and language development; legislation; research; assessment; diagnosis; behavioural management; instruction strategies; evaluation and counselling. For each of these categories, subcompetencies were also prepared, including, for example, under speech and language development the recognition of normal developmental patterns; knowledge of empirical research in language acquisition; the effects of psycho- and sociolinguistic factors on the communication process; differentiation between culturally desired linguistic conventions and deviant language and the aetiologies and remedial techniques in connection with the latter; dealing with school personnel to implement suitable instructional programmes and developing programmes for the bilingual handicapped child.

In Europe training of professionals in contact with bilingual-bicultural disabled people lags far behind even the modest aim of these proposals. An urgent need alongside expansion of research projects in the area, to extend our knowledge of appropriate diagnostic and remedial strategies, and to stipulate the branches of development that must be pursued in furthering this knowledge, is to train workers involved in what is known to date to be sound practice. A closer coordination and cooperation between clinic, school, academic interests and the target population needs also to be fostered. This coordination is often tenuous enough for monolingual disordered, but in view of the added difficulties for client and remediator alike in the bicultural context, constant liaison between all departments concerned becomes a priority. So also does increasing access to services and resources available, both by the publication of the aims and functions of various agencies to the ethnic minority communities and by the removal of barriers to the ethnic minority family in utilising the health and educational system. This demands an awareness of their needs and the adaptability and adjustment necessary to fulfil them.

Conclusion

Given the current state of knowledge, definitive answers to the many questions raised by the subject of remediation with (potentially) bilingual, language-disordered children cannot be offered. At present only partially informed recommendations can be made pending advances and confirmation of these views through future investigations. It has been argued that the basic principles of language remediation need not be different between monoglots and bilinguals, in so far as in the acquisition of language(s) they pass through the same stages, generate the same errors, and, with both of them, proficient use of at least one language is the goal. This is not to say that special linguistic difficulties would not arise in bilingual settings. Unacceptable code-mixing, possible *inter*language interference, semilingualism and (first) language loss (q.v.) are all real enough problems. Most differences, however, would appear to centre round non-linguistic criteria related to therapy outcome – for example, sociocultural considerations, and in the added decisions which have to be met regarding which language(s) should be the medium for therapy and how, when and where they should be employed. The significance of these factors is in serious need of validation through future research to establish their relevance to intervention strategies. Better intervention will only result following further insight into diagnostic and other evaluative procedures and into the process of the bilingual's language development.

However, by far the biggest obstacle remaining to progress and fairness in the field is the ignorance that often leads to prejudice through active blocking and passive indifference. This often denies recognition of the wishes and requirements of ethnic minorities and even more so of the handicapped within these communities. The last few decades have finally seen an increased academic and pedagogical interest in these groups of people, following years if not centuries of misguided attitudes to bilingualism and bilinguals. We still have a long way to travel to find the answers to all the remaining burning questions and further research and experience in this field is needed to achieve our objectives. Certainly it would be a shame, if having found answers, the favourable social-political atmosphere for the achievement of remedial objectives did not exist.

11 BILINGUAL EDUCATION. PROBLEMS AND PRACTICES

Arturo Tosi

Introduction

During the past fifteen years the presence of ethnic groups in North American and Australian societies, as well as the recent movement of rural population into industrialised Northern European countries, has caused considerable debate on the effectiveness of monolingual education for a bilingual population. In particular discussions have focused on the linguistic and educational impact of the monolingual and monocultural curriculum on linguistically and culturally diverse young people. One common objective of this debate has been the improvement of the academic performance of bilingual children born to immigrant or minority populations. Their massive school failure brought to general attention a number of social, cultural and economic problems; in particular the fact that their education was provided in a medium different from their first language and, often, from that of their community life.

In the late 1960s professional studies began to investigate the effectiveness of the monolingual curriculum and of linguistic compensatory measures for children whose mother tongue was different from that of the native, indigenous population. The alternative provision suggested consisted of a system offering simultaneous teaching in both the school language and the child's mother tongue: the two languages being referred to as those of the 'majority' (or L2) and the 'minority' groups (or L1). By the end of the 1970s several major national and international projects had emerged and most urban authorities in multi-ethnic localities had acquired experience in planning and evaluating pilot schemes concerned with the L1 of the im/migrant child. In the meantime scholars have amassed considerable data and experience. Their attention mainly focused on two separate, although interdependent, fields of inquiry. The first concerned the language attitude and use on the part of the bilingual communities and the changes undergone in the new environment. The second concentrated on the educational measures required to overcome monolingual schooling in the *majority* language and to create better learning opportunities for the *minority* bilingual child. Exposed to this academic debate, stimulated by the pronouncements of international organisations and pressurised by new political events in rapidly changing multi-ethnic societies, many countries eventually acknowledged the existence of a 'problem'. Initially seen as a question of linguistic adjustment, later discussed in connection with national trends in ethnic relations, the issue of minority children's bilingualism was soon assessed as an issue pertaining to the policies as well as the politics of education. Failure, it was suggested, does not result from a deficit dimension of a child's bilingual state, but from conditions of structured inequity inherent in the education system. In particular when the school assumes the monolingual majority child as the rule against which the bilingual minority child is found to be different, the normal measure of equal treatment does not, in fact, realise the purported principle of equal opportunity. The reaction against these normal 'compensatory' measures of monolingual schooling (and the concept of deficit, which the majority society considered inherent in the conditions of bilingual children) gradually provided new educational rationales to justify a number of reforms envisaging some form of L1 instruction alongside the child's L2 development (see Tosi, 1982c).

The aim of this chapter is not only to survey the research literature concerned with the assessment of bilingual programmes and their relevance in the education of the bilingual child. It also attempts to distinguish the theoretical from the contextual factors which have made controversial the evaluation of such educational measures in different national and societal contexts. In particular this study aims to focus on two aspects which have recently attracted the attention of language scholars. The first aspect concerns the relationship between the features of community bilingualism and the aims of the bilingual programme. The second aspect involves the relationship between societal bilingualism and the organisation of the bilingual curriculum.

The Relationship Between Community Diglossia and the Child's Early Bilingualism

In recent discussion on bilingualism it has become more customary to refer to 'bilingualism' as such when the focus is on an individual's abilities in two languages (Swain and Cummins, 1979); while 'diglossia' refers, instead, to a community's use of more than one language (Ferguson, 1959; Gumperz, 1962). A landmark distinction of the two concepts is Fishman's (1967) definition of their relationship in the different forms that it appears to be available to different speech-communities: individual bilingualism, which may or may not imply the officially recognised existence, or status, of two languages at community level (i.e. with and without diglossia); and two community languages (diglossia) which may or may not involve community members' bilingualism. The distinction introduced by Fishman between bilingualism, considered as a characterisation of individual linguistic behaviour, and diglossia as a pattern of linguistic organisation at community level, was initially discussed in relation to multilingual contexts (i.e. with monolingual individuals in a community essentially diglossic or, vice versa, with bilingual individuals in an essentially monoglossic community). However, later in the 1970s, when discussions on societal bilingualism began to question the impact, treatment and future of im/migrant populations, together with the current models of ethnic relations, Fishman's theoretical framework was adopted to assess the linguistic state of im/migrant communities in monolingual multi-ethnic societies. In a study on educational policies on migrant languages Verdoot (1977) indicates and discusses three possible relationships.

The first combination of bilingualism with diglossia implies that the im/migrants have achieved a balanced development of their infragroup and intergroup community speech that elicits full access to the repertoires of the language of the new/host country without detriment to the language of their ethnic origin. Typically such balance relies on strong attitudes of loyalty to and protection of the minority's compartmentalised community life; something which an ethnic group can only achieve through a full involvement in the majority's life, not only in linguistic, but also in economic and political terms. Two other combinations, however, appear to be more common in im/migrant communities: diglossia without bilingualism and bilingualism without diglossia. The former occurs when access to the new or host country's language is restricted. The reason for this according to Verdoot (1977) does not generally lie with the host country's authorities, but, rather, with conditions of spatial and social segregation by the migrants themselves. However, in cases when the host society stands firmly on the provisional nature of foreign labour and the principle of its rotation, several authors report that forced-segregation social policies can be found to shape school linguistic policies (Abadan-Unat, 1975; Fishman, 1977a; Tosi, 1979b and Skutnabb-Kangas, 1981). The last combination, bilingualism without diglossia, is certainly the most common relationship in immigrant communities. In the first generation the two languages show a degree of compartmentalisation, but the second generation, bilingual at an early age, becomes irreversibly monolingual under the pressure of the 'other tongue' which tends to displace the mother-tongue (see the surveys by Swain and Cummins, 1979 and by Tosi, 1979c).

This phenomenon has been shown to have two major implications: one social, one individual. On a social level, where one generation's language provides the limited data for the succeeding generation's grammar-building process, progressive changes in norms and meaning lead inevitably to the extinction of the minority language in the family and the community (Saltarelli and Gonzo, 1977 and Saltarelli, 1983). At the individual level, most investigators in assessing children's L1 have indicated that inconsistent linguistic models in the family, lack of reinforcement of accepted norms in the community and exclusion from exposure to the standard language are responsible for weakening children's L1 development (Rado, 1974; Skutnabb-Kangas, 1977; Tosi, 1979c). The conclusion of all these studies is that these conditions affect, in turn, acquisition and performance in L2; therefore the L1 development of bilingual children needs to be reinforced and supported by the school. These arguments, the evidence on which they are based, and the recommendations which follow, will be discussed in the section on 'The role of education in the child's bilingual development'.

However, the question of why the L1 of children who at home speak a language different from that used in the school needs support requires some clarification. First of all, the fact that the particular conditions of their language development weaken performance in L1, should not be confused with characteristics inherent in early bilingualism *per se*. Instead their poor L2 performance should be related to the particular features of language exposure and language infrastructures in homes and communities characterised by conditions of diglossia without bilingualism, and more often, bilingualism without diglossia. Secondly, and subsequently, lower academic performance by bilingual children in L1 programmes compared to that of their contemporary monolinguals depends, to a certain extent, on the cultural and emotional difficulty of coping with two languages (Lewis, 1970); but, to a much larger extent, results from children's seclusion from models of the standard language and from the fact that they are taught and tested in a variety of the minority language different from that spoken in the home (Tosi, 1979a, 1982a, 1983a).

Environmental conditions which depend on the particular degree of assimilation of a speech community in the majority environment and which can be described within the relationship between community diglossia and the child's early bilingualism have, of course, important educational implications. Although these questions have been amply discussed by scholars at the level of linguistic performance in both L1 and L2 (see the review by Swain and Cummins, 1979), they have attracted thus far only little interest on the part of programme planners in connection with the design of instructional and testing instruments. One recent study, however, has attempted to map some factors relevant to the construction of L1 teaching material in bilingual programmes (Tosi, 1982a). The study suggests that initial competence in L1 of children learning their mother-tongue in an L2 environment characterised by either bilingualism without diglossia, or diglossia without bilingualism, may depend on three major variables: (1) the degree of exposure to the L1 in the community; (2) the extent of use in the household; (3) the distance between the variants of L1 spoken in the household and that taught in the programme.

The Role of the Environment in the Maintenance of the Minorities' Languages

Community language-learning involves a process which is neither typical of an L2 acquisition nor of L1 development. It is useful to recall that Paulston (1975), using Gaarder's distinction between 'folk bilingualism' and 'elitist bilingualism', sharply differentiated this type of learning ('folk bilingual education') from the L2 instruction of 'elitist bilingual education'. The latter, she maintained, is the privilege of well-educated middle-class members of most societies, whilst the former is intended to cater for the ethnic groups within a single state who have to 'become bilingual involuntarily, in order to survive'. The distinction is an important one, as it shows that when the home language is valued and supported by the community, its literacy encouraged in the home, for this privileged group early L2 instructions and bilingual education has never been a problem. These children do well academically whether they are educated predominantly in the mother-tongue or in the second language (see also Swain and Cummins, 1979). Whilst for ethnic groups the linguistic models provided by the household and the support made available by the neighbourhood largely depend on the assimilatory pressure exercised by the dominant group on the community facilities and on the individuals' motivation for language maintenance. In particular, the degree of exposure to L1 in the community and the extent of its use in the household depend on the level of the group's linguistic homogeneity and its assimilation in the majority environment.

Exposure to the minority language in the neighbourhood and community accounts for the development of language infrastructures allowing for interaction between the adult members of the ethnic group. These must be confined to well-defined functions protected and compartmentalised within the minority community life and linguistically safeguarded by caretaker groups of teachers, speakers and writers. Their channels are usually community organisations, clubs, societies as well as libraries, newspapers, TV and radio programmes which circulate and broadcast social as well as official documents in the community language. The relevance of this infrastructure in the maintenance of the ethnic language at the community level is manifold and has direct implications for the stabilisation of compartmentalised roles and linguistic repertoires governing the relationship between diglossia and bilingualism. At the individual level, exposure to this linguistic network can promote the development of coordinated bilingualism, thus avoiding interferences between repertoires, loss of vocabulary, confusion between registers leading irreversibly to the group linguistic assimilation. Deprived of these external conditions of reinforcement, the minority language can gradually decay to a level of repetitive, descriptive jargon, tied to informal situations of domestic communication. The group's language loyalty will naturally suffer from the decline of its status and in particular will affect the first generation's desire to maintain it and the second generation's motivation to develop it.

The above conditions of more or less stabilised diglossia in the neighbourhood naturally affect family bilingualism and in particular the adult's interaction with the children. Often one finds that the new generation's use of the mother-tongue is confined predominantly to passive use. Moreover when the linguistic repertoires are not sufficiently compartmentalised – due to the limited sources of exposure in the community – languages begin to influence each other phonetically, morphologically and lexically. Such borrowings affecting the use of the minority language in the family might lead to discontinuous development of the child's vocabulary and restrict its repertoire to a limited range of domains.

These phenomena of language dominance and interference have, of course, a major influence on parental confidence in their medium of communication with the children. They may seriously affect their success in linguistic intervention and guidance with the child. Accurate descriptions of such attitudes (see Linguistic Minority Project Team, forthcoming) can show complex and varied mechanisms of interaction in different households within the same community or even within the same family (with older and younger children). However, since they largely depend on the level of the community's linguistic assimilation, which in turn derives from the duration of the group's settlement, its size and distribution, their major patterns tend to constitute features common to the whole community.

The third factor to be considered in the assessment of L1 development in young bilinguals is *the distance between the variety spoken in the household and the variety of instruction and testing* (often the national standard of the country of origin). This point, which has thus far attracted very little attention, has often been underestimated by policy planners as well as programme evaluators (Tosi, 1982a). It seems, however, to be a crucial one when it concerns groups who have emigrated under economic pressure from rural communities to industrialised societies, which in fact makes up the vast majority of immigrant population from the Southern regions of America and Europe to their Northern countries. In those regions where poor industrialisation and slow urbanisation have preserved large agricultural communities, a complex situation of national linguistic diversity has often survived. Many of these countries that have ignored their domestic linguistic diversity, due to lack of sensitivity to language problems or deliberate discriminatory policies (Mioni and Arnuzzo-Lanszweert, 1979), are precisely those which have offered mass unemployed labour to Northern European and American industrialised societies (Tosi, 1982c).

People who have emigrated from situations of multilingualism concealed by nationalistic linguistic homogeneity were linguistically different and discriminated against in their own country before they became so in the new or host society. For these groups, policies involving the 'teaching of the mother tongue of the country of origin' (see the ambiguous phrasing of the EEC directive, 1977), may just fail to do justice to the bilingualism of their children, when their L1 is assumed to be the national standard of the country of origin (Tosi, 1978). The outcome may in fact disappoint communities and educators who, expecting the benefits of better learning opportunities from L2 development through L1 reinforcement and literacy, are actually implementing a much more complex process of learning which involves simultaneously:

the language of the country of origin	=	L3 =	language of instruction and literacy (but not exposure)
the language of the host/new society	=	L2 =	language of exposure, literacy and instruction taught to speakers of
the rural dialect	=	L1 =	the native language of the home and immediate environment but used neither for instruction nor literacy

Naturally in the case of some minority groups, competence in the vernacular may not impede natural intelligibility of the standard or other privileged codes chosen for instruction: it could only marginally decrease accuracy in relation to production skills. But for other communities, when the term vernacular actually refers to idioms based on a system substantially different from that of the national standard, more time, training and sophisticated strategies may be required even to produce oral intelligibility. For example, multidialectism in Italy involves so-called 'dialects' found to be as distant from each other and the standard as two independent languages of the same family (i.e. Portuguese and Romanian, see Pellegrini, 1960). Naturally a delay in transferring oral L1 skills into literacy in L3 makes the problem of reading and writing in the community language much more serious than a question of accuracy. In this case one could hardly define the advantage of early literacy in the 'mother-tongue' as one anchored in a native competence.

This important question pertaining to the multidialectal composition of the minority group, together with the factors related to the stabilisation of diglossia in its neighbourhood, are fundamental in the identification of the young child's bilingualism in relation to his/her community language, whether this is the mother-tongue learnt in the home, a variety spoken in the neighbourhood or the national standard different from both. As all of these issues are closely linked to the arguments of *why* and *how* L1 should be taught to young bilingual children, they will be further discussed in connection with the controversial role of the school in the child's bilingual development.

The Role of Education in the Child's Bilingual Development

To the question 'why should such children be taught their mother-tongue alongside the language of their school and society?' there are various answers. The findings of several studies show it to be a twofold problem. Following Fishman's analysis of societal bilingualism and language change in multilingual communities (1972), some scholars relate 'mother-tongue teaching' in school programmes to new linguistic objectives and to forward-looking social policies. Such studies tend to focus on minority languages' new status and their culture-carrying nature in a society looking for alternatives to the melting pot hypothesis. Others question the effectiveness of compensatory education operated by the majority group: this happens when the latter ignores the minority children's linguistic repertoire, and attempts to adapt them to the sociocultural model of the dominant group.

The two positions are obviously interdependent. Both groups of scholars in criticising monolingual schooling and compensatory education, have used research findings interchangeably. The issue of cultural pluralism and minority groups' language rights constitute the central arguments for mother-tongue teaching among those scholars questioning the philosophy of assimilation-oriented monolingual/monocultural education systems. A classic review of the arguments for and against language rights of im/migrant groups can be found in Kloss (1971). He discusses four main arguments for assimilation (e.g. the tacit contracts, the 'take and give', the anti-ghettoisation and the national unity theories) and examines seven arguments in support of the opposite view (i.e. im/migrants have the right to retain and cultivate their own languages). He then distinguishes between promotion-oriented and tolerance-oriented language rights, concluding that im/migrant groups can lay no claims to promotion-oriented measures unless they prove that their desire to keep their languages alive lasts more than a generation. On the other hand, Kloss admits that there may be pedagogical arguments in favour of promotion-oriented measures: elementary schools can use the pupils' L1 to speed up their eventual assimilation.

Verdoot (1977), analysing Kloss's arguments, adopts Fishman's (1967) distinction between bilingualism and diglossia. Bilingualism without diglossia, he points out, tends to be a transitional stage, since it provides no support for the development of second-generation bilingualism. When, instead, maintenance support is provided for the mother-tongue, the community speech develops into bilingualism with diglossia: the only desirable relationship, according to Verdoot. But Verdoot also warns that not all such support provision is designed to maintain their languages. This point is spelt out by many other scholars who, attempting to analyse the social implications of bilingual programmes, have considered whether they promote language maintenance or language shift.

Those particularly concerned with the linguistic needs of young bilingual children emphasise emotional disturbances and slow linguistic and cognitive development of pupils whose mother-tongue is different from the school language. In 1970 Lewis, drawing on the work of Luria (1932) and Spoerl (1946), maintained that bilingual children's emotional conflicts result from tensions between linguistic settings. Their emotional maladjustment is not so much generated by the complexity of thinking and speaking in two languages, as by cultural conflict. During the 1970s many studies reported advantages in early rather than late L2 learning (Burstall, 1975; Macnamara, 1976; Titone, 1977). Two Finnish scholars, Skutnabb-Kangas and Toukomaa (1976), however, taking Malmberg's point (1971a) that most of this argument is based on the imitative character of early language-learning, claimed that early instruction in L2 threatens L1 development and hinders cognitive growth. They base their argument on the theories of psychologists such as Vigotsky (1962) and Luria and Yudovich (1956), who maintain that verbal communication between child and adult has the double function of regulating further external communication and reorganising the child's mental process and cognitive abilities. Since im/migrants' children lack satisfactory preschool verbal interaction with adults, the two Finns maintain the L2 teaching should be delayed until cooperation between cognitive functioning and linguistic operation can be minimised. In consequence they argue that when academic performance and linguistic skills of young bilingual children of im/migrants are compared with those of monolinguals, the low scores attained in both languages could be attributable to conditions of semilingualism, i.e. when someone can 'function' in two languages, but is not really proficient in either (Hansegård, 1968). A number of subsequent experiments and studies have attempted to establish correlations between the sociolinguistic conditions considered typical of 'semilingualism' respectively with competence in L1 (Jaakkola, 1974) in L2 (Wrede, 1972) and school achievements (Hansegård, 1968 and Tenerz, 1966). All these studies indicate consistently the inadequacy of monolingual L2 education and support the hypothesis that instruction and literacy in L1 could counteract the negative effect of semilingualism.

The linguistic conditions of the Finnish communities in Sweden were increasingly to attract the attention of linguists and educators as it became more widely recognised that the origin of the children's low academic achievement and worse social opportunities was the inadequacy of the language provision offered by the school. As Malmberg put it, as early as 1971 (1971b) 'they are linguistically and consequently intellectually handicapped by their bilingual status, not because of bilingualism as such, but on account of their lack of primary education in the language they spoke in their homes as children'. Loman (1974) further explains that 'semilingualism has been used as a term for the type of faulty linguistic competence which has especially been observed in individuals, who have since childhood had contact with two languages without sufficient or adequate training and stimulation in either of the two languages' (translation by Paulston, 1975).

So far, however, the notion of semilingualism has proved difficult to quantify in linguistic terms. As reported in Paulston (1975), some scholars have pointed to the vagueness of definition and to the inadequacy of measurement (Loman, 1974; Pinomaa, 1974; Koskinen, 1974 and Nordin, 1974; all in Loman, 1974). Paulston, when reviewing these works, points out that all of the 'anti-semilingualism' studies have dealt with post-puberty subjects; although she cannot find evidence that the level of mother-tongue competence is unsatisfactory for the functional needs in the diglossic community, she accepts that one should consider the possible effect of semilingualism on early schooling, given the fact that these children have never been exposed to a fully developed language, or as Hymes put it 'they give up one language before they learn a second' (Hymes, 1974a, cited in Paulston, 1978).

In the second half of the 1970s the Finnish-speaking communities of Sweden provided the area for a substantial exploration and assessment of the conditions of semilingualism. A large-scale study supported by UNESCO and carried out by Skutnabb-Kangas and Toukomaa (1976) (see also Toukomaa and Skutnabb-Kangas, 1977) was to reinforce these arguments. The project involved a sample of 687 Finnish pupils in 171 comprehensive school classes in Sweden. In the evaluative report the two investigators explain:

> the purpose of the study was to determine the linguistic level and development in both mother tongue and Swedish (L_2) of Finnish migrant children attending Swedish comprehensive schools. Above all attention was paid to the interdependence between skills in the mother tongue and Swedish, i.e. the hypothesis was that those who have best preserved their mother tongue are also best in Swedish. Related to this question, the significance of age at which the child moved to Sweden was also determined. Do those who received a firm grounding in their mother tongue by attending school in Finland have a better chance of learning Swedish than those who moved to Sweden as pre-scholars? A second important problem was

> the achievement of Finnish pupils in Swedish-language schools. How do Finnish migrant pupils do in theoretical and what might be called practical subjects? Does one's skill in the mother tongue have any effect on the grade given in a Swedish-language school or on other school achievement? (Skutnabb-Kangas and Toukomaa, 1976).

The findings of the study showed that: (1) language skills of all of these students measured by standardised tests were considerably below Finnish and Swedish norms; (2) a strong correlation existed between the development of the mother-tongue prior to contact with Swedish and later proficiency in that language. In particular the experiment demonstrated that with L1 reinforcement by education (i.e. children who migrated at the age of 10 after being schooled in Finland), mother-tongue maintenance close to the level of Finnish monolingual competence was possible, as well as a development of L2 skills close to those of Swedish monolinguals. However, children who moved to Sweden at an early age (7, 8 or younger) were most likely to achieve low levels of literacy in both languages. On the basis of these findings Skutnabb-Kangas and Toukomaa argue that (1) L1 development has functional significance in the acquisition of L2 and that the mother-tongue should be developed and reinforced by the school; (2) where only low competence in the mother-tongue is attained, this will limit the development of competence in L2, so affecting cognitive functioning and academic achievement and justifying Lambert's description of 'semilingualism' as a subtractive type of bilingualism (1977).

The findings of psychological studies on individual bilingualism and education together with the more sociologically oriented arguments from the debate on societal bilingualism and language change in multilingual communities provided the main guidelines to set up the criteria for the identification, design and evaluation of different models of bilingual education. Subsequently two main aspects of bilingual-bicultural programmes were identified by researchers as most relevant in evaluating the implications for both the child and the community. One includes the role of L1 in the curriculum (how, to what extent and with what objective it is taught). The other focuses on the impact of minority language maintenance on the wider sociocultural context. Accordingly researchers in this area have devised a typology to group the different programmes into categories. Most of them seem to accept that there can be two major orientations in such models:

1. *Compensatory/transitional*. The L1 (minority or marked language) is used to enable the poor speaker or non-speaker of the L2 (majority or unmarked language) to master subjects until skills in L2 are developed. The outcome is transitional bilingualism for the child and assimilation for the minority group.
2. *Language maintenance*. The marked language is emphasised and introduced as a more stable medium of instruction, while the unmarked language is introduced gradually, until they both become media of instruction for all subjects. The outcome is balanced bilingual coordinate competence in individuals and cultural pluralism in the community. The minority group preserves its own language and becomes diglossic for compartmentalised intragroup and intergroup purposes.

Several studies, however, when reviewing this typology recognise the possible dangers inherent in the first and second models in certain socio-political contexts (see Spolsky, 1974). The first, Fishman (1977b) points out, designed to be compensatory for the child, is imposed and absorptive. The second, he warns, though fostering societal bilingualism and cultural pluralism, can become separative. This can happen when the majority of the population is not interested in learning the marked language or when provision is offered to encourage segregation and repatriation, e.g. teaching in Turkish to children of Turks in Bavarian schools (Fishman, 1977a). The solution suggested by Verdoot (1977) of 'bilingualism with diglossia' resulting from language maintenance might therefore produce segregation. Fishman proposes as an alternative relationship, double diglossia, where the school-related language of one group is the home and neighbourhood language of the others and vice versa. Such a programme in the long term is then neither absorptive nor separative, but an additive and enriching one for both the marked and the unmarked populations involved (*enrichment oriented*).

Further appraisals and evaluations of different bilingual programmes can be found in discussions on the threshold hypothesis in Cummins (1976), Paulston (1977), Toukomaa and Skutnabb-Kangas (1977) and Swain and Cummins (1979). Their arguments suggest that a bilingual curriculum should incorporate so-called language shelter programmes which delay the teaching of L2 until a sufficient level of competence in L1 is reached to guarantee the achievement of the threshold level. This is justified by the fact that the school should (1) compensate for the im/migrant parents' limited opportunities for providing stimuli and models and (2) reinforce interaction between linguistic operations and cognitive functions. Such aid could only be given by a system (1) offering im/migrants' children intensive L1 teaching from preschool onwards, and (2) delaying L2 teaching until there are well-developed L1 structures on which both L2 and subjects in L2 can be anchored.

Since the late 1970s the debate on the child's bilingualism and bilingual education has progressed considerably from the previous decades and its more recent developments seem to focus on three areas. These are: (1) the definition of the im/migrant child's bilingual state; (2) the evaluation of the impact of his/her bilingualism on the school and overall society; and (3) the design of instructional materials suitable for the particular conditions of mother-tongue development in the context of second-language learning. The second and third areas will be discussed in the following sections. The first, which relates directly to the definition and educational treatment of 'bilingualism', leads to much discussion on the controversial notion of 'semilingualism'. Brent-Palmer (1979), in a paper entitled 'A Sociolinguistic Assessment of the Notion "Im/migrant Semilingualism" from a Social Conflict Perspective' strongly condemns the new theory likely to present the language of these children within a new deficit perspective and to elicit further compensatory approaches. Unfairly, it would seem, she directs her criticism to those who adopt the notion of 'semilingualism', although they have always stressed that the deficit dimension of semilingualism is not inherent in the im/migrant children's bilingualism. Rather it is based on the monolingual school that utilises the monolingual majority child as the rule against which the minority child is found to be different (or semilingual) (Skutnabb-Kangas and Toukomaa, 1980). However, some of the facts cited by Brent-Palmer are worth consideration especially in relation to the likelihood of exploiting mother-tongue provision in bilingual programmes as a final therapeutic formula of 'subtractive bilingualism'. In particular she refers to situations where instruction in the standard variety of the im/migrants' children's mother-tongue may pose even more problems than education via the second language. Many im/migrants, she points out, do not speak a standard variety of their mother-tongue before migrating (see also Bubenik, 1978; Canale and Mougeon, 1978; Karttunen, 1977; and Tosi, 1981 and 1983a). Even more phenomena of language contact tend to produce frequent morphological and/or syntactic generalisations and simplifications, further complicating the use of such languages in vernacular education.

Indeed, it would seem that a clarification of these issues (not only within a theoretical-cognitive perspective, but also within an applied pedagogical one) needs to be advanced for a better understanding of 'semilingualism' or 'subtractive bilingualism' at the level of curriculum development, material design and teacher training. In particular it is significant that those education systems in which a positive approach towards the linguistic diversity of their schools and communities has produced a definite policy of promotion of community languages, have been the first to pose the most relevant questions and to attempt to find some answers. Ultimately their concerns relate to the fundamental question of how community language teaching should differ from the teaching of the same language as an L2 to foreign learners or as an L1 to monolingual natives. Here the problem of the bilingual child's initial competence in his/her mother-tongue immediately appears to be one of extreme relevance to course planners, classroom teachers as well as materials designers.

Mother-tongue Teaching in the Context of Second-language Learning

Community language teaching for bilingual children has not only brought about a considerable revolution in the area of language pedagogy but has also opened up a challenging field of new theoretical questions and practical problems for language planners, curriculum and materials designers as well as teacher trainers. In particular, in programmes of community language the problem of initial competence becomes one of paramount importance. This has, however, so far produced among the practitioners no more than the awareness that it involves a learning process which is typical neither of L1 development nor of L2 acquisition (see the report by Bourne and Trim, 1980). In a study which follows my work for the EEC/Bedford project of mother-tongue development by Italian and Punjabi bilingual children in English schools (Tosi, 1983a) and in discussions within the National Congress on Languages in Education (Tosi, 1982a) I have attempted to conceptualise a framework for the analysis of this learning process. In particular I have attempted to map all possible factors relevant to the learner, the target language and the environmental learning conditions, which make the specific process of mother-tongue development in the context of second-language learning different, respectively, from L1 development and L2 acquisition. In a subsequent investigation the relevance of this set of variables was tested in view of a definition of the bilingual child's initial competence in his/her community language. This latter field study was commissioned by the Catholic Education Office of Victoria, Australia, which was primarily concerned with the design and evaluation of reading and instructional materials, linguistically relevant to teaching Italian as a community language to young bilinguals in Australia (Tosi, 1982b). The working hypothesis was that only by investigating those variables, could one formulate assumptions about community language learning by bilinguals (*mother-tongue development in the context of second-language learning*) different, respectively, from the assumptions currently accepted for L1 and L2 learning. In the former case, in fact, the learner's initial competence is assumed as nil. In the second case it is referred to as 'native', which often tends to be taken as synonymous with 'total mastery'. In reality in most learning environments things are not so straightforward. In the study which provided the theoretical framework for the investigation of Italian spoken by Italians in Australia, I have tried to present visually, in an integrated structure, the interconnection between the social and linguistic conditions of different language learning processes (Tosi, 1982b). These processes include: (1) monolingual development for monolingual children; (2) bilingual development for mono/bilingual children; (3) monolingual development for bidialectal children; (4) mother-tongue development in the context of second-language learning.

An ideal model describing a language-learning process is probably most easily thought of as similar to a multi-tiered cylinder. The bottom layer contains variables relative to the language spoken in the home and the immediate family environment; the middle layer contains factors relative to language infrastructure and sources of exposure in the community; and the top layer contains components of the school curriculum designed to develop its pupils' linguistic resources to meet the standards of language competence demanded by society. The dimension of such standards is represented by the size of the top circle of the cylinder in Figure 11.1. Since the achievement of these standards is the goal of any linguistic education policy, it is clear that the greater the fulfilment of the volume of each of the three layers sustaining the top, the firmer the support given to the child's language development.

The four different learning processes mentioned above can be visualised in the four cylinders shown in Figure 11.2 associated in three cases with other shapes representing the different distributions of variables relevant to different monolingual and bilingual learning processes:

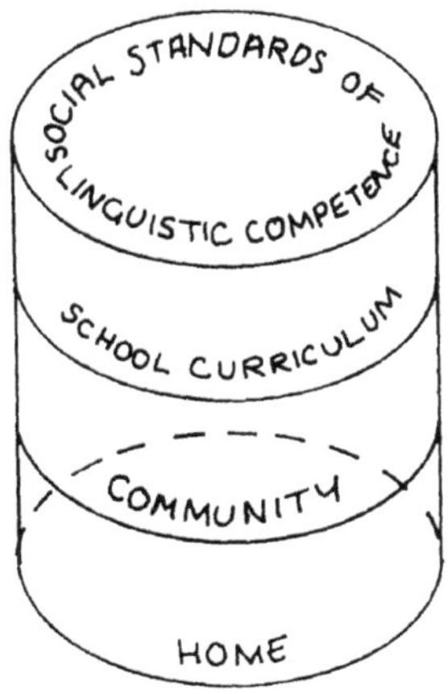

Figure 11.1

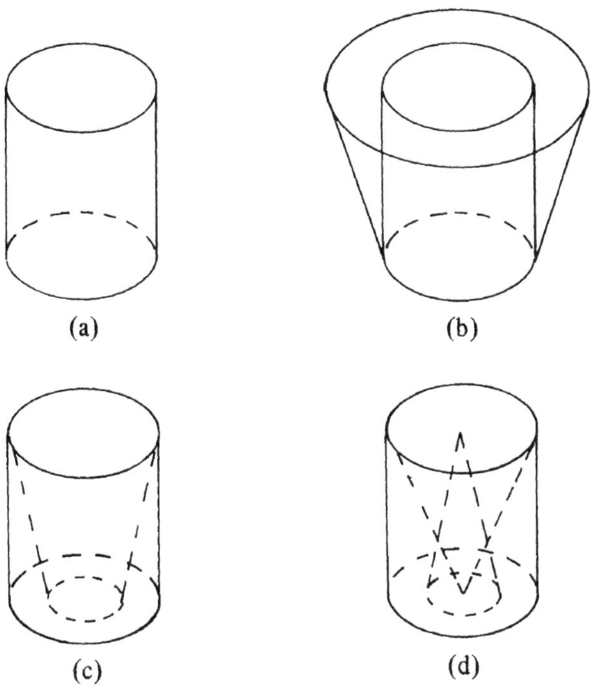

Figure 11.2

Figure 11.2(a) represents the typical situation of monolingual children from a family background where the standard language is spoken and linguistic guidance support is provided by the parents and the immediate circle of neighbours and peers. They are exposed to the same language in an environment rich in sources of exposure to selected and sophisticated patterns of linguistic interactions. The school's role is to reinforce and organise their language competence to meet the demands of the curriculum. Their overall monolingual development in the standard language is protected, and directed towards the achievement of the standards demanded by their monolingual school and society; standards that they are most likely to meet as a result of concomitant situations converging their language development into a channel (the cylinder) which concentrates their efforts on the fulfilment of the academic and social goals created by that society.

Figure 11.2(b) represents the more privileged conditions of bilingual development for children from a solid mono/bilingual background, who benefit from bilingual education in the mother-tongue with a high-status foreign/second language. The figure consists of a cylinder corresponding to the situation described in the previous section, where the base may or may not include a bilingual situation at home. The volume enclosed between the cylinder and the truncated cone surrounding it represents the extra measures taken within the three adjoining sections to maintain and develop a bilingualism with no detriment to a solid linguistic experience and education in the mother-tongue. The linguistic standards demanded by society in one's national/standard language (also the pupil's mother-tongue) are achieved (top circle), and at the same time there is a chance to achieve bilingualism in another high-status language (as represented by the wider circle of the truncated cone), and to be able to operate linguistically in a multi/inter/national dimension.

Figure 11.2(c) represents the far more common situation of monolingual schooling for a child who lives in a bidialectal family and environment. The standards of linguistic competence demanded by society in the national language remain the same, as represented by the top circle, whilst the truncated cone enclosed in the cylinder represents the limited family/environmental support available to the child for the development of his/her competence in the standard language. In particular, a limited family training in the standard, poor sources of exposure to that language in the community and the inability of the school to cope effectively with bidialectal children all result in dispersion of efforts (represented in Figure 11.2(c) by the section of volume between the cylinder and truncated cone). This happens when the school and society value only competence in the standard and disregard or even penalise any other dialect.

Figure 11.2(d) represents the process identified as *'mother-tongue development in the context of second-language learning'*, one typical of minority pupils learning their first language in a multi-ethnic society. The top circle, representing the standards of linguistic competence necessary to achieve equal social opportunities, remains the same in a society with a multilingual population – but a monolingual policy – as in a society with a monolingual population (compare Figure 11.2(a)). The achievement of such standards, however, becomes even more difficult for linguistically diverse children, than in the situation described in Figure 11.2(c). In fact, their point of departure – the family support in relation to the majority (L2) language – is almost non-existent (which in the figure is represented by the apex of the inverted cone). Facilities for L2 development increase in the environment and the school, although they form a much poorer complex of environmental situations in comparison to those in the three other cases. The mother-tongue, instead, starts from a more favourable position – as represented by the base of the other cone – although it might often be a rural or contact dialect of little use outside the community and stigmatised even in the homeland. Its development might originally benefit from a rich infrastructure within the family and neighbourhood, but in later life, not reinforced by full conditions of exposure, the mother-tongue might develop only within restricted domains. At school, with the exception of those countries which have adopted a bilingual education policy, the mother-tongue might occupy a minimal portion of the timetable or even by confined outside the monolingual school.

A comparison between the two shapes representing two situations of bilingual development (including one form of bilingualism valued and another disdained by society) shows that, in the first case, the original cylinder is surrounded by additional volume, as in Figure 11.2(b), whilst in the other cylinder, Figure 11.2(d), a portion of volume has been subtracted. This accords with Lambert's (1977) distinction between 'additive' and 'subtractive' bilingualism. He says that in the first situation 'the bilingual is adding another socially relevant language to his/her repertoire of skills at no cost to his/her L_1 competence'; in the second, 'the bilingual's competence in his/her two languages at any point is likely to reflect some stage in the "subtraction" of L_1 and its replacement by L_2'. The latter case, Lambert further comments, is typical of 'many ethnic minority groups who, because of national educational policies and social pressures of various sorts, are forced to put aside their ethnic language for a national language'. As these speakers may be characterised by less than native-like competence in both languages, the studies reported above have investigated their conditions in terms of 'double-semilingualism' or 'semilingualism'.

Conclusions

Since the late 1950s considerable research literature has developed covering a wide range of aspects of language competence and language education for normally developing bilingual children. Three main areas of questions have developed. The first includes sociolinguistic issues concerning the definition and description of early bilingual abilities with specific attention to the role of the family and the neighbourhood in the development of preschool competence in both L1 and L2. The second incorporates the arguments which make a case for bilingual education as well as the discussions on its advantages compared with those made available by monolingual schooling. The third is concerned with the sociopolitical evaluation of different bilingual reforms as reflections of different national language policies. The scholars' aim is to assess the changes of language education as part of the curriculum development within different education systems in general and *vis-à-vis* policies for a culturally and socially diverse population in particular. Within the first field of enquiry research has consistently shown that the linguistic conditions inherent in the diglossic minority community (i.e. the family and neighbourhood) are responsible for weakening L1 development in the child, who may then appear linguistically handicapped in the resulting competition with the monolingual pupil. In consequence investigators tend to view the treatment of the minority child's L1 by the school as an expression of the society's attitude towards ethnic bilingualism and minorities' languages.

Exposed to this professional debate many industrialised countries have introduced bilingual reforms including programmes of 'mother-tongue' or 'community-languages' teaching. As for the evaluation of this provision, however, educationalists do not seem to have reached full agreement. In particular, much discussion has centred on whether the school *ought* to, and whether its curriculum actually *can* provide as good a command of the L1 (the minority language) as children would attain in a school in the country of origin, and as good linguistic skills in the L2 (the majority language) as the monolingual indigenous children achieve in their L1. In this case, however, writers seem to be divided by specific professional practices as well as fundamental political perspectives.

In the area of professional practices more evidence, which must be derived from diverse national contexts, is needed to reinforce the view that the curriculum can actually adopt L1 instruction with no detriment to L2 development. This would finally settle the controversy of *whether* and *how* bilingual education *per se* can lead to societal bilingualism by fostering individual language competence and community language confidence.

Beyond strictly professional pedagogical matters, other important issues have divided scholars as well as practitioners. These controversies involve the evaluation of practices adopted by certain education systems towards pupils who, while developing their bilingualism as normal children, are made to appear culturally and linguistically disabled by the system itself, when put in competition with native monolinguals. Discussion of this issue in different countries, however, has shown the incomparability of school attitudes as well as linguistic objectives of bilingual programmes in different national contexts. Bilingual competence can in fact be differently used: to avoid cultural assimilation or to equip against linguistic isolation in the new/host society. In situations with a highly mobile population it can also help educational reintegration in the country of origin in case of return. Naturally the different types of linguistic competence needed to meet such diverse social objectives can not be realistically achieved simultaneously by any general formula of bilingual programme. Therefore specific programmes of L1 taught alongside L2 must require different approaches, priorities, instruments and further, in some cases, they may involve different varieties of the same 'community language'. Since all these questions pertain to the sphere of linguistic emancipation of social groups, which in different systems is operated by diverse means of social and economic control, they should also be analysed as political issues. Their political nature derives, in fact, from the societal interpretation of *what the value of bilingualism is* rather than from the professional assessment of *what bilingual competence is and how it can be improved*. The latter two are typical questions belonging to a professional linguist's perspective. Although this perspective is important it is not, however, the only relevant one when discussing the future of children caught between the normal development of their bilingualism and its, often, abnormal treatment by a monolingual society.

BIBLIOGRAPHY

Abadan-Unat, N. (1975), 'Educational Problems of Turkish Migrants' Children', *International Review of Education*, XXI, 2, 309-22.

Abudarham, S. (1976), 'A Study of the Word-familiarity and Age-of-Acquisition Variables of a Word List', compiled as a potential vocabulary test for bilingual children. Unpublished M.Sc dissertation, University of London.

— (1980a), 'Problems of Assessing the Linguistic Potential of Children with Dual Language Systems and their Implications for the Formulation of a Differential Diagnosis', in M. Jones (ed.), *Language Disability in Children* (MTP, Lancaster), pp. 231-46.

— (1980b), 'The Role of the Speech Therapist in the Assessment of Language Learning Potential and Proficiency of Children with Dual Language Systems or Background', *J. Multiling. Multicult. Devel.*, 1, 3, 187-206.

— (1982), 'Communication Problems of Children with Dual-Language Systems or Backgrounds: to Teach or to "Therapise"', *Int. Schools J.*, 3, Spring, 43-54.

Adams, M. (1978), 'Methodology for Examining Second Language Acquisition', in E. Hatch (ed.), *Second Language Acquisition* (Newbury House, Rowley, Mass.), pp. 277-96.

Adler, S. (1981), *Poverty Children and Their Language: Implications for Teaching and Treating* (Grune-Stratton, New York).

Aitchison, J. (1972), 'Mini-malapropisms', *Brit. J. Discord. Comm.*, April, 38-43.

Albrow, K.H. (1972), *The English Writing System: Notes Towards a Description*, Schools Council Programme in Linguistics and English Teaching: Papers Series *II*, vol. 2 (Longman, London).

Anderson, A. (1979), 'Survival of Ethnolinguistic Minorities: Canadian and Comparative Research', in H. Giles *et al.* (eds), pp. 67-85.

Anderson, E. (1979), 'The Reading Behaviour of a Group of Children of Families of West Indian Origin', unpublished MPhil thesis, University of Nottingham, School of Education.

— (1981), 'Dialect and Text', in L.J. Chapman (ed.), *The Reader and the Text* (Heinemann Educational Books, London), pp. 99-105.

Anderson, J. (1976), *Psycholinguistic Experiments in Foreign Language Testing* (University of Queensland Press, St Lucia).

— (1982), 'The Measurement of the Perception of Cohesion: a Second Language Example', paper presented at the International Reading Association Ninth World Congress on Reading, Dublin, July.

Anthony, A., Bogle, D., Ingram, T.T.S. and McIsaac, M.W. (1971), *The Edinburgh Articulation Test* (Livingstone, Edinburgh).

Baetens-Beardsmore, H. (1980), 'Bilingualism in Belgium', *J. Multiling. Multicult. Devel.*, 1, 2, 145-54.

— (1982), *Bilingualism: Basic Principles* (Tieto, Clevedon).

Ball, M.J. and Munro, S.M. (1981), 'Language Assessment Procedures for Linguistic Minorities: an Example', *J. Multiling. Multicult. Devel.*, 2, 231-41.

Ballard, C. (1979), 'Conflict, Continuity and Change: Second Generation South Asians', in V. Saifullah-Khan, pp. 109-30.

Barik, H. and Swain, M. (1976), 'A Longitudinal Study of Bilingual and Cognitive Development', *Int. J. Psychology*, 11, 251-63.

Basso, K. (1970), 'To Give up on Words. Silence in Western Apache Culture', *S.W.J. of Anthrop*, 26, 213-30.

Bates, E. (1976), *Language and Contexts: The Acquisition of Pragmatics* (Academic Press, New York).

— and MacWhinney, B. (1982), 'Second Language Acquisition from a Functionalist Perspective; Pragmatic, Semantic and Perceptual Strategies', in H. Winitz (ed.), *Conference on Native and Foreign Language Acquisition* (New York Academy of Sciences, New York).

Bellin, W. (1983), 'Welsh Phonology in Acquisition', in M.J. Ball and G.E. Jones (eds), *Welsh Phonology: Selected Readings* (University of Wales Press, Cardiff).

Benjamin, L. and Pratt, R. (eds) (1975), *Transcultural Counselling: Needs, Programs, Techniques* (Ann Arbor, Michigan ERIC Clearinghouse on Counselling and Personnel Services).

Ben-Zeev, S. (1972), 'The Influence of Bilingualism on Cognitive Development-and-Cognitive Strategy', unpublished PhD, University of Chigaco.

— (1975), *The Effect of Spanish-English Bilingualism in Children from Less-privileged Neighborhoods on Cognitive Development*, Research Report to HEW Nat. Inst. Child Health and Human Devel., USA.

— (1976), 'What Strategies do Bilinguals Use in Preventing their Languages from Interfering with Each Other, and what Effect does this have on Non-language Tasks?', *Papers and Reports on Child Language Development*, 12, Stanford University, Department of Linguistics.

—(1977), 'The Influence of Bilingualism on Cognitive Strategy and Cognitive Development', *Child Development*, 48, 1009-18.

Berdan, R. (1981), 'Black English and Dialect-Fair Instruction', in N. Mercer (ed.), pp. 217-36.

Bergin, V. (1980), *Special Education Needs in Bilingual Programs*, Office of Bilingual Education. Eric Doc. ED 197 527.

Bernal, E. (1975), 'A Response to Educational Uses of Tests with Disadvantaged Subjects', *Amer. Psy.*, 30, 93-5.

Berry, J. (1966), 'Temne and Eskimo Conceptual Skills', *Int. J. Psy.*, 1, 207-29.

Berry, M. (1980), *Teaching Linguistically Handicapped Children* (Prentice-Hall Inc., Englewood Cliffs, New Jersey).

Bever, T. (1970), 'The Cognitive Basis for Linguistic Structures', in J. Hayes (ed.), *Cognition and the Development of Language* (Wiley, New York).

Blom, J. and Gumperz, J. (1972), 'Social Meaning in Linguistic Structures: Code Switching in Norway', in J. Gumperz and D. Hymes (eds), *Directions in Sociolinguistics* (HRW, New York), pp. 407-34.

Bloom, L., Lightbown, P. and Hood, L. (1975), 'Structure and Variation in Child Language', *Monog. Soc. for Res. in Child Devel.*, 40, (Serial 160).

— and Lahey, M. (1978), *Language Development and Language Disorders* (Wiley, New York).

Blum-Kukla, S. (1982), 'Learning to Say what you Mean in a Second Language: A Study of the Speech Act Performance of Learners of Hebrew as a Second Language', *Applied Linguistics*, 3, 29-59.

Bourhis, R. (1979), 'Language in Ethnic Interaction: a Social Psychological Approach', in H. Giles *et al.*, pp. 117-41.

Bourne, R. and Trim, J.L.M. (1980), 'European Commission Mother Tongue and Culture Pilot Project', unpublished report of the Colloquium on the Bedford Mother Tongue Project held at the Cranfield Institute of Technology, 24-27 March.

Bowerman, M. (1973), *Early Syntactic Development: A Cross Linguistic Study with Special Reference to Finnish* (CUP, Cambridge).

Brent-Palmer, C. (1979), 'A Socioloinguistic Assessment of the Notion "Im/migrant Semilingualism" from a Social Conflict Perspective', *Working Papers on Bilingualism*, 17, 135-80.

Brown, R. (1973), *First Language* (Penguin, Harmondsworth).

Bruck, M., Lambert, W.E. and Tucker, G.R. (1974), 'Cognitive Consequences of Bilingual Schooling: The St Lambert Project Through Grade 7', *Lang. Learn.*, 24, 183-204.

— Tucker, G.R. and Jakimik, F. (1975), 'Are French Immersion Programs Suitable for Working Class Children?', in W. Von Raffler Engel (ed.), *Prospects in Child Language* (Mouton, The Hague).
— Lambert, W.E. and Tucker, G.R. (1976), 'Cognitive and Attitudinal Consequences of Bilingual Schooling: The St Lambert Project Through Grade Six, unpublished research report, McGill University.
— (1978), 'The Suitability of Early French Immersion Programs for the Language-disabled Child', *Canadian J. of Education*, 3, 45-72.
— (1982), 'Language-impaired Children's Performance in an Additive Bilingual Education Program', *Applied Psycholing.*, 3, 45-61.
Bruner, J. (1966), 'On Cognitive Growth' in J. Bruner, R. Olver and P. Greenfield (eds), *Studies in Cognitive Growth* (Wiley, New York).
Bubenik, V. (1978), 'The Acquisition of Czech in the English Environment', in M. Paradis (ed.), *Aspects of Bilingualism* (Hornbeam Press Inc., Columbia, South Carolina), pp. 3-12.
Burling, R. (1959), 'Language Development of a Garo and English-Speaking Child', *Word*, 15, 45-68.
Burstall, C. (1975), 'Factors Affecting Foreign Language-learning: a Consideration of some Recent Findings', *Language-Teaching and Linguistics: Abstracts*, 8.
Burt, M. and Dulay, H. (1980), 'On Acquisition Orders', in S. Felix (ed.), *Second Language Development* (Narr, Tubingen, Germany), pp. 265-327.
Canale, M. and Mougeon, R. (1978), 'Problèmes Posées par la Mesure du Rendement en Français des Elèves Franco-Ontariens', *Working Papers on Bilingualism*, 16, 92-100.
— and Swain, M. (1980), 'Theoretical Bases of Communicative Approaches to Second Language Teaching and Testing', *Applied Linguistics*, 1, 1-47.
— (1983), 'From Communicative Competence to Communicative Language Pedagogy', in J. Richards and R. Schmidt (eds), *Language and Communication* (Longman, New York), pp. 2-27.
Cancel, C.A. (1976), 'Lisping in Spanish: a Defect or a Dialectal Trend?', *Int. J. Oral Myology*, 2, 4, 94-7.
Canfield, D.L. (1981), *Spanish Pronunciation in the Americas* (University of Chicago Press, Chicago).
Carpenter, P.A. and Just, M.A. (1977), 'Integrative Processes in Comprehension', in D. La Berge and S.J. Samuels (eds), *Basic Processes in Reading: Perception and Comprehension* (Lawrence Erlbaum Associates, Hillsdale, N.J.), pp. 217-41.
Carrasco, R. (1979), *Expanded Awareness of Student Performance: A*

Case Study in Applied Ethnographic Monitoring in a Bilingual Classroom (SEDL, Austin, Texas).

Carringer, D.C. (1974), 'Creative Thinking Abilities of Mexican Youth: The Relationship of Bilingualism', *J. Cross-cultural Psych.*, 5, 492-504.

Carrow, E. (1971), 'Comprehension of English and Spanish by Preschool Mexican-American Children', *Mod. Lang. J.*, 55, 371-80.

Cazden, C. (1972), *Functions of Language in the Classroom* (Teachers College Press, New York).

Celce-Murcia, J. (1978), 'The Simultaneous Acquisition of English and French in a Two-Year-Old', in E. Hatch (ed.), *Second Language Acquisition* (Newbury House, Rowley, Mass.), pp. 38-53.

Chapman, L.J. (1982), *Reading Development and Cohesion* (Heinemann Educational, London).

Chapman, R. (1981), 'Exploring Children's Communicative Intents', in J. Miller, pp. 111-36.

Charrow, V. (1974), *Deaf English – An Investigation of the Written English Competence of Deaf Adolescents*, Tech. Report 236, Inst. for Math. Studies in Soc. Sci., Stanford University.

Cheng, C., Brizendine, E. and Oakes, J. (1979), 'What is 'an Equal Chance' for Minority Children', *J. Negro Educ.*, 48, 3, 267-87.

Ching, D.C. (1976), *Reading and the Bilingual Child* (International Reading Association, Newark, Delaware).

Chinn, K. (1980), 'Assessment of Culturally Diverse Children', *Viewpoints in Teach. Learn.*, 56, 1, 50-63.

Chomsky, N. and Halle, M. (1968), *The Sound Pattern of English* (Harper Row, New York).

Christensen, E. (1975), 'Counselling Puerto Ricans: Some Cultural Considerations', *Personnel and Guidance J.*, 53, 5, 349-56.

Clark, M.M. (1980), *Reading Difficulties in Schools* (Heinemann Educational, London; first published by Penguin, 1970).

Clay, M.M. (1972), *Concepts about Print Test: Sand* (Heinemann Educational, Auckland).

—— (1979), *Concepts about Print Test: Stones* (Heinemann Educational, Auckland).

—— (1981a), *Reading: the Patterning of Complex Behaviour* (Heinemann Educational, London; first published, 1973).

—— (1981b), *The Early Detection of Reading Difficulties: A Diagnostic Survey with Recovery Procedures* (Heinemann Educational, London; first published, 1972).

Cleary, T., Humphreys, L., Kendrick, S. and Wesman, A. (1975),

'Educational Uses of Tests with Disadvantaged Students', *Amer. Psy.*, 30, pp. 15-41.

Coard, B. (1971), *How the West Indian Child is made ESN in the British School System* (New Beacon Books, London).

Compton, C. (1980), *A Guide to 65 Tests for Special Education* (Pitman Learning, Inc., CA).

Cook-Gumperz, J. and Corsaro, W. (1975), *Social-Ecological Constraints on Children's Communicative Strategies* (Xerox).

Corder, S.P. (1971), 'Idiosyncratic Dialects and Error Analysis', *IRAL*, 9, 2, 147-60.

— (1981), *Error Analysis and Interlanguage* (OUP, Oxford).

Cornejo, R. (1973), 'The Acquisition of Lexicon in the Speech of Bilingual Children', in P. Turner (ed.), *Bilingualism in the Southwest* (University of Arizona Press, Tucson), pp. 67-93.

Cowan, J.R. and Sarmed, Z. (1976), 'Reading Performance of Bilingual Children According to Type of School and Home Language', *Working Papers on Bilingualism*, 11, ED 129057.

Cromer, R. (1970), 'Children are Nice to Understand: Surface Structure Clues to Recovery of a Deep Structure', *Brit. J. Psy.*, 61, 397-408.

Crystal, D., Fletcher, P. and Garman, M. (1976), *Grammatical Analysis of Language Disability* (Arnold, London).

— (1980), *Introduction to Language Pathology* (Arnold, London).

— (1981), *Clinical Linguistics* (Springer, Wien; New York).

— (1982), *Profiling Linguistic Disability* (Arnold, London).

Cummins, J. and Gulutsan, M. (1974), 'Some Effects of Bilingualism on Cognitive Functioning', in S. Carey (ed.), *Bilingualism, Biculturalism and Education* (Univ. Alberta Press, Edmonton).

— (1976), 'The Influence of Bilingualism on Cognitive Growth: a Synthesis of Research Findings and Explanatory Hypothesis', *Working Papers on Bilingualism*, 9, 1-43.

— and Mulcahy, R. (1978), 'Orientation to Language in Ukranian-English Bilingual Children', *Child Development*, 49, 1239-42.

— (1979), 'Linguistic Interdependence and the Educational Development of Bilingual Children', *Rev. Educ. Res.*, 49, 222-51.

— (1980), 'Psychological Assessment of Immigrant Children. Logic or Intuition', *J. Multiling. Multicult. Devel.*, 1, 2, 97-111.

— (1980a), 'The Construct of Language Proficiency in Bilingual Education', in J. Alatis (ed.), *Georgetown University Round Table on Languages and Linguistics* (Georgetown University Press, Washington, DC), pp. 81-103.

— (1981), 'The Role of Primary Language Development in Promoting

Educational Success for Language Minority Students', in *Schooling and Language Minority Students: A Theoretical Framework* (Office of Bilingual Bicultural Education, California State Department of Education, Sacramento, California).

Cziko, G. (1975), 'The Effects of Different French Immersion Programs on the Language and Academic Skills of Children from Various Socioeconomic Backgrounds', MA thesis, Department of Psychology, McGill University.

Daitchman, M. (1976), 'Reading and Listening Comprehension of Fluent Bilinguals in the Native and Second Languages', unpublished manuscript, Concordia University.

Daniels, J. and Houghton, V. (1972), 'Jensen, Eysenck and the Eclipse of the Galton Paradigm', in K. Richardson *et al.* (eds), *Race, Culture and Intelligence* (Penguin Harmondsworth), pp. 68-80.

Darley, F. and Siegel, G. (1979), *Evaluation of Appraisal Techniques in Speech and Language Pathology* (Addison-Wesley, Phillipines).

Day, R., Gallimore, R., Tharp, R., Chan, K. and Connor, M. (1978), 'Order of Difficulty of Standard Eng. Grammatical Features among Cultural Minority Groups in the US', *Anthrop. Educ. Qtly.*, 9, 3, 181-95.

— (1981), 'Silence and the ESL Child', *TESOL Qtly.*, 15, 35-9.

Deignan, M. and Ryan, K. (1979), *Annotated Bibliog. of Bilingual Teaching* (New England Teacher Corps Network. Eric Doc. ED 196 178).

Derrick, J. (1977), *Language Needs of Minority Group Children* (NFER, Windsor).

de Villiers, P. and de Villiers, J. (1979), *Early Language* (Fontana/Open Books, London; Harvard UP, Camb., Mass.).

Diamond, E. (1981), *Item Bias Issues: Background Problems, and Where we are Today* (AERA, Los Angeles).

Donahue, M.L. (1981), 'Requesting Strategies of Learning Disabled Children', *Applied Psycholing*, 2, 213-34.

Donaldson, M. and Reid, J. (1982), 'Language Skills and Reading: a Developmental Perspective', in A. Hendry (ed.), *Teaching Reading: the Key Issues* (Heinemann Educational, London), pp. 1-14.

Downing, J. and Thackray, D.V. (1975), *Reading Readiness* (Hodder and Stoughton, London).

Dulay, H. and Burt, M. (1974), 'Natural Sequences in Child Second Language Acquisition', *Language Learning*, 24, 37-53.

— and Burt, M. (1974a), 'Errors and Strategies in Child Second Language Acquisition', *TESOL Qtly.*, 8, 2, 129-36.

— and Burt, M. (1974b), 'You Can't Learn Without Goofing', in J. Richards (ed.), *Error Analysis: Perspectives on Second Language Acquisition* (Longman, London), pp. 95-123.

—, Hernández-Chávez, E. and Burt, K. (1978), 'The Process of Becoming Bilingual', in S. Singh *et al.* (eds), *Diagnostic Procedures in Hearing, Speech and Language* (University Park, Baltimore), pp. 251-304.

Dumont, R. (1972), 'Learning English and How to be Silent: Studies in Sioux and Cherokee Classrooms', in C. Cazden *et al.* (eds), *Functions of Language in the Classroom* (Teachers College Press, New York).

Duran, R. (1981), *Hispanic Research SIG Presentation* (AERA, Los Angeles).

Edgerton, R. (1979), *Mental Retardation* (Fontana/Open Books, London).

Edwards, J. (1977), 'Students' Reactions to Irish Regional Accents', *Lang. Sp.*, 20, 280-6.

Edwards, J. (1979), *Language and Disadvantage*, (Arnold, London).

— (1981), 'Context of Bilingual Education', *J. Multiling. Multicult. Devel.*, 2, 1, 25-44.

Edwards, P. (1978), *Reading Problems: Identification and Treatment* (Heinemann Educational, London).

Edwards, V.K. (1979), *The West Indian Language Issue in British Schools* (RKP, London).

— (1980), 'Black British English, a Bibliographical Essay on the Language of Children of West Indian Origin', in *SAGE Race Relations Abstracts*, vol. 5, nos. 3/4, 1-25.

— (1981), *Language Variation in the Multicultural Classroom* (Centre for the Teaching of Reading, University of Reading, England).

Eliás-Olivares, L. (1976), 'Language Use in a Chicano Community: a Sociolinguistic Approach', *Working Papers in Sociolinguistics*, 30, Feb. (SW Educ. Devel. Lab., Austin).

Elliot, A. (1981), *Child Language* (CUP, London).

Erickson, F. (1981), *Hispanic Research SIG Presentation* (AERA, Los Angeles).

Ervin-Tripp, S. (1981), 'Social Process in First- and Second-Language Learning', in H. Winitz (ed.), *Native Language and Foreign Language Acquisition* (New York Academy of Sciences, New York), pp. 33-47.

European Community Council (1977), Council Directive on the Education of Children of Migrant Workers, 25 July, 77/486/EEC.

Evard, B. and Sabers, D. (1979), 'Speech and Language Testing with Distinct Ethnic-racial Groups. A Survey of Procedures for Improving

Validity', *J. of Speech and Hearing Disorders*, 44, Aug., 255-70.

Eysenck, H. (1973), *The Inequality of Man* (Maurice Temple-Smith, London).

Fair Play for Children (1982), *All Children Play, Background Information on Play in Multiracial Britain* (248 Kentish Town Road, London NW5).

Fantini, A. (1976), *Language Acquisition of a Bilingual Child* (Experiment Press, Brattleboro, Vermont).

— (1978), 'Bilingual Behaviour and Social Cues: Case Study of Two Bilingual Children', in M. Paradis (ed.), *Aspects of Bilingualism* (Hornbeam Press, Columbia, South Carolina).

Fathman, A. (1975), 'The Relationships Between Age and Second Language Productive Ability', *Language Learning*, 25, 245-53.

Favreau, M., Komoda, M.K. and Segalowitz, N. (1980), 'Second Language Reading: Implications of the Word Superiority Effect in Skilled Bilinguals', *Canadian J. Psy.*, 4, 370-81.

— and Segalowitz, N. (1982), 'Second Language Reading in Fluent Bilinguals', *Applied Psycholing*. 3, 329-41.

Ferguson, C. (1959), 'Diglossia', *Word*, 15, 325-40.

Fillmore, L.W. (1976), 'The Second Time Around: Cognitive and Social Strategies in Second Language Acquisition', unpublished doctoral dissertation, Stanford University.

— (1979), 'Individual Differences in Second Language Acquisition', in C. Fillmore, D. Kempler, W. Wang (eds), *Individual Differences in Language Ability and Language Behaviour* (Academic Press, New York), pp. 203-41.

— (1983), 'The Language Learner as an Individual: Implications of Research on Individual Differences for the ESL Teacher', in M. Clarke and J. Handscombe, *On TESOL '82: Pacific Perspectives on Language Learning and Teaching* (Teachers of English to Speakers of Other Languages, Washington, DC), pp. 157-73.

Find-a-Story (Penguin Books, Harmondsworth) (no date).

Fishman, J.A. (1967), 'Bilingualism With and Without Diglossia; Diglossia With and Without Bilingualism', *J. Social Issues*, 23, 2, 29-38.

— (1972), *Languge and Nationalism* (Newbury House, Rowley, Mass.).

— (1977a), 'Bilingual Education for the Children of Migrant Workers: the Adaptation of General Models to a New Specific Challenge', in M. De Grève and E. Rossell (eds), *Problèmes linguistiques des enfants des travailleurs migrants* (10e Colloque de l'AIMAV en collaboration avec la Commission des Communeautés Européennes,

Brussels: AIMAV, Didier).
— (1977b), 'The Social Science Perspective: Keynote', in J.A. Fishman (ed.), *Bilingual Education: Current Perspectives*, vol. 1 (Center for Applied Linguistics, Arlington, Va.), pp. 1-49.
— (1980), 'Bilingualism and Biculturalism as Individual and Societal Phenomena', *J. Multiling. Multicult. Devel.*, 1, 1, 3-15.
Fitzgerald, M. and McLachlan, I. (1978), 'Immigrants: Do We Understand Them Enough to Help Them', *Nursing Mirror*, Aug. 17, p. 34.
Fitzpatrick, F. (1981), 'The Language Question in the Multicultural School', *Multiracial Education*, 10, 1, 3-20.
Fletcher, P. and Garman, M. (eds) (1979), *Language Acquisition* (CUP, Cambridge).
Francis, H. (1975), *Language in Childhood* (Elek, London).
Fraser, W. (1978), 'Speech, Language Development of Children with Down's Syndrome', *Devel. Med. Child Neurol.*, 20, 106.
— and Grieve, R. (eds) (1981), *Communicating with Normal and Retarded Children* (Wright, Bristol).
Gal, S. (1979), *Language Shift: Social Determinants of Language Change in Bilingual Austria* (Academic Press, London).
Garcia, E. and Aguilera, R. (1979), 'Language Switching During Mother-Child Bilingual Interaction', in R. Anderson (ed.), *The Acquisition and Use of Spanish and English as First and Second Languages* (Teachers of English to Speakers of Other Languages, Washington, DC), pp. 164-73.
— (1980), 'Bilingualism in Early Childhood', *Young Children*, 35, 4, 52-66.
Gardner, P.L. (1978), 'Difficulties with Illative Connectives in Science amongst Secondary School Students', *The Austl. Science Teachers J.*, 24, 3, 23-30.
Genesee, F., Tucker, G.R. and Lambert, W.E. (1975), 'Communication Skills of Bilingual Children', *Child Development*, 46, 1013-18.
— (1976), 'The Role of Intelligence in Second Language Learning', *Lang. Learn.*, 26, 267-80.
— and Chaplin, S. (1976), *Evaluation of the 1974-75 Grade II French Immersion Class* (Department of Psychology, McGill University).
— and Stefanovic, B. (1976), *Evaluation of the 1975-76 Grade II French Immersion Class* (Instructional Services, The Protestant School Board of Greater Montreal).
— (1978), 'A Longitudinal Evaluation of an Early Immersion School Program', *Canad. J. of Education*, 3, 31-50.
— (1983), 'Bilingual Education of Majority-language Children: The

Immersion Experiments in Review', *Applied Psycholing*., 4, 1-46.

Gerken, K. (1978), 'Performance of Mexican-American Children on Intelligence Tests', *Exceptional Child*, 44, 6, 438-43.

Gibson, E.J. and Levin, H. (1975), *The Psychology of Reading* (MIT Press, Cambridge, Mass).

Gil, R. (1981), 'Puerto Rican Mothers' Cultural Attitudes Toward the Use of Mental Health Services', in H. Martinez (ed.), pp. 49-60.

Giles, H. (ed.) (1977), *Language Ethnicity and Intergroup Relations* (Academic Press, London).

— and Saint-Jaques, B. (eds) (1979), *Language and Ethnic Relations* (Pergamon, London).

Glaser, G. (1982), 'Critical Periods in Brain Development Related to Behaviour', in J. Apley *et al.* (eds), *One Child* (Heinemann Medical, London), pp. 54-74.

Goldman, R. and Fristoe, M. (1972), *Test of Articulation* (American Guidance Services, Inc., Circle Pines, Minn.).

Goodacre, E.G. (1976), 'Assessment', in C. Longley (ed.), *Teaching Young Readers* (BBC, London), pp. 91-109.

— (1979), *Hearing Children Read* (Centre for the Teaching of Reading, University of Reading, Reading).

Goodman, K.S. and Goodman, Y.M. (1977), 'Learning about Psycholinguistic Processes by Analyzing Oral Reading', *Harvard Educ. Rev*., 47, 3 Aug., 317-85.

— (1982), Workshop, United Kingdom Reading Association 19th Course and Conference, Newcastle Polytechnic, Newcastle-upon-Tyne.

Gray, T. (1978), *Skills and Competencies Needed by the Bilingual-Bicultural Special Educator* (CAS, Va.).

Greenfield, P.M. (1966), 'On Culture and Conservation', in J. Bruner, R. Olver and P.M. Greenfield (eds), *Studies in Cognitive Growth* (Wiley, New York).

Grieve, R. and Hoogenraad, R. (1976), 'On Using Language if you Don't have Much', in R. Wales and E. Walter (eds), *New Approaches to Language Mechanisms* (North Holland), pp. 1-28.

— and Hoogenraad, R. (1979), 'First Words', in P. Fletcher *et al.* (eds), pp. 93-104.

— (1981), 'Observations on Communication Problems in Normal Children' in W. Fraser *et al.*, pp. 65-83.

Grill, J. and Bartel, N. (1977), 'Language Bias Tests: ITPA Grammatic Closure', *J. Learn. Disabil*., 10, 4, 229-35.

Grunwell, P. (1982), *Clinical Phonology* (Croom Helm, London).

Gumperz, J.J. (1962), 'Types of Linguistic Communities', *Anthrop. Ling.*, 4, 1, 28-40.

— (1964), 'Speech Variations and the Study of Indian Civilisation', in D. Hymes (ed.), *Language in Culture and Society* (Harper Row, New York), pp. 416-23.

— (1977), 'Sociocultural Knowledge in Conversational Inference', in M. Saville-Troike (ed.), pp. 191-212.

— (1982), *Discourse Strategies* (CUP, Cambridge).

Gunzburg, H. (1975), *Progress Assessment Chart of Social and Personal Development* (SEFA, Stratford-upon-Avon).

Haberland, H. and Skuttnab-Kangas, T. (1979), 'Political Determinants of Pragmatic and Sociolinguistic Choices', *Rolig-Papir*, 17, Roskilde Universitetscenter.

Hahn, J. and Dunston, V. (1974), 'Bilingualism and Individualised Parent Education, an Organic Approach to Early Childhood Education', *California J. of Educ. Res.*, 25, 5, 253-60.

Hakes, D.T. (1982), 'The Development of Metalinguistic Abilities: What Develops?', in S. Kuczaj (ed.), *Language Development, vol. II: Language, Thought and Culture* (Erlbaum Hillsdale, NJ).

Halliday, M. (1978), *Language as Social Semiotic* (Arnold, London).

— and Hasan, R. (1980), 'Text and Context', *Sophia Linguistica Working Papers in Linguistics No. 6* (Sophia University Linguistic Institute, Tokio).

Hansegård, N.E. (1968), *Tvaspråkighet eller halvspråkighet?* (Alddusserien 253, Stockholm, 3rd edn).

Harris, S. (1978), 'Traditional Aboriginal Education Methods Applied in the Classroom', *Austl. J. Early Childhood*, 3, 17-23.

Harrison, G. and Piette, A. (1980), 'Young Bilingual Children's Language Selection', *J. Multiling. Multicult. Devel.*, 1, 3, 217-30.

Hatch, E. (1983), *Psycholinguistics: A Second Language Perspective* (Newbury House, Rowley, Mass.).

Haugen, E. (1953), *The Norwegian Language in America*, vols 1, 11 (Univ. Penn. Press, Philadelphia).

— (1954), 'Review of Weinreich, *Language in Contact*', *Language*, 30, 380-8.

Hecht, B. and Mulford, R. (1982), 'The Acquisition of a Second Language Phonology: Interaction of Transfer and Development Factors', *Applied Psycholing.*, 3, 313-28.

Hegarty, S. and Lucas, D. (1978), *Able to Learn? The Pursuit of Culture Fair Assessment* (NFER, Windsor).

Henderson, P. (1976), 'Class Structure and the Concept of Intelligence', in R. Dale, G. Esland, M. McDonald (eds), *Schooling and Capitalism* (RKP, London).

Henley, A. (1979), *Asian Patients in Hospital and at Home* (Kings Fund/Pitman Medical, London).

— (1980), 'Health in Other Cultures', *GP*, 15 Feb., 52-4.

HMSO (1981), *West Indian Children in Our Schools* (Her Majesty's Stationery Office, London).

Herman, D. (1979), *Identification of Bilingual Handicapped Students* (Pensylvania Resources and Information Center, Eric Doc. ED. 169 709).

Hickman, M. (1982), 'The Development of Narrative Skills: Pragmatic and Metapragmatic Discourse Comprehension', doctoral dissertation, University of Chicago.

Howard, D. (1982), 'Pitfalls in the Multicultural Diagnostic/Remedial Process. A Central American Experience', *J. Multiling. Multicult. Devel.*, 3, 1, 41-6.

Hoyle, E. (1980), 'Additional Problems faced by Hearing-impaired Children of Asian Parentage', *J. Brit. Ass. Teach. Deaf.*, 4, 1, 15-20.

— (1981), 'Deaf Children in (Asian) Immigrant Families in the UK', *Talk*, 99, 18-20.

Hudson, R. (1980), *Sociolinguistics* (CUP, London).

Hudson, W. (1967), 'The Study of the Problem of Pictorial Perception Among Unacculturated Groups', *Int. J. Psy.*, 2, 89-107.

Hunter, E. (1977), *Reading Skills: a Systematic Approach* (Council for Educational Technology, London).

Hyman, L.M. (1975), *Phonology: Theory and Analysis* (HRW, New York).

Hymes, D. (1971), *On Communicative Competence* (University of Pennsylvania Press, Philadelphia).

— (1974), *Foundations of Sociolinguistics* (University of Pennsylvania Press, Philadelphia).

— (1974a), 'Speech and Language: On the Origins and Foundations of Inequality Among Speakers', in M. Bloomfield, *et al.* (eds), *Language as a Human Problem* (W.W. Norton, New York), pp. 45-71.

Ianco-Worrall, A. (1972), 'Bilingualism and Cognitive Development', *Child Development*, 43, 1390-400.

Imedadze, N. (1967), 'On the Psychological Nature of Child Speech Formulation Under Conditions of Exposure to Two Languages', *Int. J. of Psy.*, 2, 129-32.

Ingram, D. (1976), *Phonological Disability in Children* (Arnold, London).

— (1979), 'Phonological Patterns in the Speech of Young Children', in P. Fletcher and M. Garman (eds).

Itoh, H. and Hatch, E. (1978), 'Second Language Acquisition: A Case Study', in E. Hatch (ed.), *Second Language Acquisition* (Newbury House, Rowley, Mass.), pp. 76-88.

Jaakkola, M. (1974), 'Den Sprakgransen Variationen: Svenska Tornedalen', in B. Loman (ed.).

Jackson, G. (1975), 'Comment on the Report of the ad hoc Committee on Educational Uses of Tests with Disadvantaged Students', *Amer. Psy.*, 30, 88-93.

Jackson, H. (1981), 'Errors of Punjabi Speakers of English', *ITL*, 54, also *CORE*, 3/3 1979 Fiche 10, D11-F7.

Jacobson, R. (1982), 'The Social Implications of Intra-sentential Code-switching', in J. Amastae and L. Eliás-Olivares (eds), *Spanish in the United States: Sociolinguistic Aspects* (CUP, Cambridge).

Jahangiri, N. and Hudson, R. (1982), 'Patterns of Variation in Tehrani Persian', in S. Romaine (ed.), pp. 49-64.

Jakobson, R. (1942), *Kindersprache, Aphasie und allgemeine Lautgesetze* (Uppsala). Translated (1968) *Child Language, Aphasia and Phonological Universals* (Mouton, The Hague).

—, Fant, C.G.M. and Halle, M. (1952), *Preliminaries to Speech Analysis* (MIT Press, Cambridge, Mass.).

James, C. (1980), *Contrastive Analysis* (Longman, Harlow).

Jeffree, D. and McConkey, R. (1976), *PIP Developmental Charts* (Hodder and Stoughton, Sevenoaks).

Jensen, S. (1972), *Educability and Group Differences* (Methuen, London).

Jespersen, O. (1922), *Language, Its Nature, Development and Origin* (Allen and Unwin, London).

Johnson, D. (1983), 'Natural Language Learning by Design: A Classroom Experiment in Social Interaction and Second Language Acquisition', *TESOL Qtly*, 17, 55-68.

Jones, D. (1951), *The Phoneme, Its Nature and Its Use* (Heffers, Cambridge).

Jones, I. (1979), 'Some Cultural and Linguistic Considerations affecting the Learning of English by Chinese Children in Britain', *Eng. Lang. Teach. J.*, 34, 1, 55-69.

Jones, R.O. (1983), 'Change and Variation in the Welsh of Gaiman, Chubut', in M.J. Ball and G.E. Jones (eds), *Welsh Phonology: Selected Readings* (University of Wales Press, Cardiff).

Karmiloff-Smith, A. (1979), 'Language Development after Five', in

P. Fletcher *et al.* (eds), pp. 307-23.

Karttunen, F. (1977), 'Finnish in America: A Case Study in Monogenerational Language Change', in B.A. Blount and M. Sanches (eds), *Sociolinguistic Dimensions of Language Change* (Academic Press, New York), pp. 21-33.

Keller-Cohen, D. (1981), 'Input from the Inside: The Role of a Child's Prior Linguistic Experience in Second Language Learning', in R. Andersen (ed.), *New Dimensions in Second Language Acquisition Research* (Newbury House, Rowley, Mass.), pp. 95-103.

Kessler, C. (1971), *Acquisition of Syntax in Bilingual Children* (Georgetown University Press, Washington, DC).

— (1976), 'Linguistic Universals in Anthropological Studies of Bilingualism', in W. McCormack and S. Wurm (eds), *Language and Man* (Mouton, The Hague), pp. 177-88.

— and Idar, I. (1977), 'The Acquisition of English Syntactic Structures by a Vietnamese Child', in C. Henning (ed.), *Proceedings of the Second Language Acquisition Forum* (University of California, Los Angeles), pp. 295-307.

— and Idar, I. (1979), 'The Acquisition of English by a Vietnamese Mother and Child', *Working Papers on Bilingualism*, 18, 65-80.

Kirk, S., McCarthy, J. and Kirk, W. (1968), *Illinois Test of Psycholinguistic Abilities* (University of Illinois Press, Urbana, Ill.).

Kloss, H. (1971), 'Language Rights and Immigrant Groups', *Int. Migration Rev.*, 5, 250-68.

Kochman, T. (1981), 'Classroom Modalities: Black and White Communicative Styles in the Classroom', in N. Mercer (ed.), pp. 96-114.

Koskinen, I. (1974), 'Svensk interferens i Torneddalsfinskan', in B. Loman (ed.).

Krashen, S. (1981), *Second Language Acquisition and Second Language Learning* (Pergamon Press, Oxford).

— (1982), *Principles and Practice in Second Language Acquisition* (Pergamon Press, Oxford).

Labov, W. (1970), 'The Study of Language in its Social Context', *Studium Generale*, 23, 66-84.

Lado, R. (1957), *Linguistics Across Cultures* (University of Michigan Press, Ann Arbor).

Lago, C. and Ball, R. (1983), 'The Almost Impossible Task: Helping in a Multi-cultural Context', *Multiracial Education*, 11, 2, 39-50.

Lambert, W.E. (1975), 'Culture and Language as Factors in Learning and Education', in A. Wolfgang (ed.), *Education of Immigrant Students* (Ontario Institute for Studies in Education, Toronto).

— (1977), 'The Effect of Bilingualism on the Individual: Cognitive and Sociocultural Consequences', in P. Hornby (ed.), *Bilingualism: Psychological, Social and Educational Implications* (Academic Press, New York), pp. 5-27.

Landry, R. (1974), 'A Comparison of Second Language Learners and Monolinguals on Divergent Thinking Tasks at Elementary School Level', *Modern Lang. J.*, 58, 10-15.

Language Support Services (1982), *Talking and Telling: Language, Stories and Games in the Multicultural Classroom* (English Language Centre, Lydford Road, Reading, England).

Lantolf, J. (1980), 'Spanish in the United States Setting: Beyond the Southwest', speech at University of Illinois at Chicago Circle conference.

Laosa, L.M. (1977), 'Historical Antecedents and Current Issues in Non-discriminatory Assessment of Children's Abilities', *School Psychol. Digest*, 6, 3, 48-56.

Lapointe, C. (1976), 'Token Test Performances by Learning Disabled and Achieving Adolescents', *Brit. J. Disord. Comm.*, 11, 2, 121-33.

Lavandera, B.R. (1981), 'Lo quebramos, but Only in Performance', in R.P. Duran (ed.), *Latino Language and Communicative Behavior* (Ablex, Norwood, NJ).

Lee, L. (1974), *Developmental Sentence Analysis* (Northwestern University Press, Evanston, Ill.).

Leonardi, M. (1981), 'Paragraph Reading and Sentence Connection in Achieving Comprehension in English as a Second Language', in L.J. Chapman (ed.), *The Reader and the Text* (Heinemann Educational, London), pp. 163-70.

Leopold, W. (1939, 1947, 1949a, 1949b), *Speech Development of a Bilingual Child*, 4 vols (Northwestern University Press, Evanston, Ill.).

Le Page, R. (1975), 'Sociolinguistics and the Problem of "Competence"', *Lang. Teach. and Ling. Abs.*, 8, 137-56.

Lerman, A. (1980), 'Improving Services to Hispanic Hearing Impaired Students', in M. Pynn, pp. 17-30.

Leudar, I. (1981), 'Strategic Communication in Mental Retardation', in W. Fraser *et al.* (eds), pp. 113-29.

Lewis, E.G. (1970), 'Immigrants – their Languages and Development', *Trends in Education*, 18, 25-32.

— (1981), *Bilingualism and Bilingual Education* (Pergamon, Oxford).

Lewycka, M., Mares, P. and Whitaker, N. (1980), *The HELP Maternity Language Course* (Leeds City Council).

Lindholm, K. and Padilla, A. (1978), 'Language Mixing in Bilingual Children', *J. Child Lang.*, 5, 327-35.

Linguistic Minorities Project Team (forthcoming), *Linguistic Minorities in England* (provisional title), (RKP, London).

Lobo, E. (1978), *Children of Immigrants to Britain* (Hodder and Stoughton, London).

Loman, B. (1974), *Språk och Samhalle, 2. Språket i Tornedalen* (CWK Gleerup Bokforlag, Lund).

Lopez-Schule, L. (1982), 'The Simultaneous Acquisition of English and Spanish', unpublished research paper, University of Texas at San Antonio.

Luetke, B. (1976), 'Questionnaire Results from Mexican-American Parents of Hearing Impaired Children in the US', *American Annals of the Deaf*, 121, 6, 565-8.

Lunzer, E.A. and Gardner, K. (1979), *The Effective Use of Reading* (Heinemann Educational/Schools Council, London).

Luria, A.R. (1932), *The Nature of Human Conflicts* (Liveright, New York; US edn, 1967).

— and Yudovich, F. (1956), *Speech and the Development of Mental Processes in the Child,* 1971 edn (Penguin, Harmondsworth).

[*Mc* is indexed as *Mac*]

Ma, R. and Herasimchuk, E. (1968), 'The Linguistic Dimensions of a Bilingual Neighbourhood', in J. Fishman *et al.*, *Bilingualism in the Barrio* (Yeshiva University, New York).

Macaulay, R. (1977), *Language, Social Class and Education: a Glasgow Study* (Edinburgh University Press, Edinburgh).

Mace-Matluck, B.J., Hoover, W.A. and Dominguez, D. (1981), *Variation in Language Use of Spanish-English Bilinguals in Three Settings (Classroom, Home and Playground): Findings and Implications* (AERA, Los Angeles), April.

McEntegart, D. and LePage, R. (1982), 'An Appraisal of the Statistical Techniques used in the Sociolinguistic Survey of Multilingual Communities', in S. Romaine (ed.), pp. 105-24.

Mackay, D., Thompson, B. and Schaub, B. (1970), *Breakthrough to Literacy: Teacher's Manual* (Longman/Schools Council, London).

MacKinnon, K. (1977), *Language, Education and Social Processes in a Gaelic Community* (RKP, London).

McLauchlin, R. (1980), 'Speech Protocols for Assessment of Persons with Limited Language Abilities', in R. Rupp and K. Stockdell (eds), *Speech Protocols in Audiology* (Grune, Stratton, New York), pp. 253-86.

McLaughlin, B. (1977), 'Second Language Learning in Children', *Psy. Bull.*, 84, 3, 438-59.

— (1978), *Second Language Acquisition in Childhood* (Erlbaum, Hillsdale, NJ).

— (1981), 'Differences and Similarities Between First and Second Language Learning', in H. Winitz (ed.), *Native Language and Foreign Language Acquisition* (New York Academy of Sciences, New York), pp. 23-32.

— (1982), *Children's Second Language Learning* (Center for Applied Linguistics, Washington, DC).

Macnamara, J. (1976), 'First and Second Language Learning: Same or Different?', *J. Educ.*, 158, 239-54.

MacWhinney, B. (1977), 'Starting Points', *Language*, 53, 152-67.

Malmberg, B. (1971a), *Språkinlärning. En Orientering och ett Debattinlägg* (Aldusserien 339, Aldus/Bonniers, Stockholm).

— (1971b), 'Applications of Linguistics', in G. Perrin and J. Trim (eds), *Selected Papers of the Second International Congress of Applied Linguistics* (CUP, London), pp. 3-18.

Marcos, L.R., Urcuyo, L., Kesselman, M. and Alpert, M. (1973), 'The Language Barrier in Evaluating Spanish-American Patients', *Archives of General Psychiatry*, 29, 5, 655-9.

Mares, P. (1981), *Background Information for Health Workers, No. 1. Vietnamese and their Health in Britain* (National Extension College, Cambridge).

Martin, F. and Hart, D. (1978), 'Measurement of Speech Thresholds of Spanish-speaking Children by non-Spanish-speaking Clinicians', *J. Speech, Hearing Disorders*, 43, 255-62.

Martinez, H. (ed.) (1981), *Special Education and the Hispanic Child. Proceedings from the Annual Colloquium on Hispanic Issues*, Clearing-house on Urban Education (Teachers College, Columbia University, Eric Doc. ED 210 404).

Meisel, J., Clahsen, H. and Pienemann, M. (1981), 'On Determining Developmental Stages in Natural Second Language Acquisition', *Studies in Second Language Acquisition*, 3, 109-35.

Mercer, J. (1976), *Labelling the Children* (NIMH, Rockville, Maryland).

— and Lewis, J. (1978), *System of Multicultural Pluralistic Assessment: Student Assessment Manual* (Psychol. Corp., New York).

— (1979), 'In Defense of Racially and Culturally non-Discriminatory Assessment', *School Psychol. Digest*, vol. 8, no. 1.

Mercer, N., Mercer, E. and Mears, R. (1979), 'Linguistic and Cultural Affiliation Amongst Asian People in Leicester', in H. Giles *et al.*

(eds), pp. 15-26.
— (ed.) (1981), *Language in School and Community* (Arnold, London).
Mikeš, M. (1967), 'Acquisition des Catégories Grammaticales dans le Language de l'Enfant', *Enfance,* 20, 289-97.
Miller, G. (1969), 'The Organisation of Memory: Are Word Associations Sufficient?', in G.A. Talland and N.C. Waugh (eds), *The Pathology of Memory* (Academic Press, New York).
Miller, J. (1981), *Assessing Language Production in Children. Experimental Procedures* (Arnold, London).
Miller, N. (1978), 'The Bilingual Child in the Speech Therapy Clinic', *Brit. J. Disord. Comm.*, 13, 1, 17-30.
Milroy, L. (1980), *Language and Social Networks* (Blackwell, Oxford).
Mioni, A. and Arnuzzo-Lanszweert, A.M. (1979), 'Sociolinguistics in Italy', *Int. J. Soc. Lang.*, 21, 81-107.
Morehead, D. (1975), 'The Study of Linguistically Deficient Children', in S. Singh (ed.), *Measurement Procedures in Speech, Hearing and Language* (University Park, Baltimore), pp. 19-53.
Morris, J. (1974), *Language in Action Resource Books* (Macmillan, London).
Morrow, K. (1977), *Techniques of Evaluation for a Notional Syllabus* (Royal Society of Arts, London).
Moseley, C. and Moseley, D. (1977), *Language and Reading among Underachievers* (NFER, Windsor).
Mowder, B. (1980), 'Strategy for the Assessment of Bilingual Handicapped Children', *Pschology in the Schools*, 17, 1, 7-11.
Mueller, D., Munro, S.M. and Code, C. (1981), *Language Assessment for Remediation* (Croom Helm, London).
Murrell, M. (1966), 'Language Acquisition in a Trilingual Environment: Notes from a Case Study', *Studia Linguistica*, 20, 9-34.
National Extension College (no date), *Lessons from the Vietnamese: a Kit for Tutors of English as a Second Language* (NEC, Cambridge).
Nelson, K. (1975), 'The Nominal Shift in Semantic Syntactic Development', *Cog. Psychology*, 7, 461-79.
Nelson-Burgess, S. and Meyerson, J. (1975), 'MIRA; A Concept in Receptive Language Assessment of Bilingual Children', *Language, Speech, Hearing Services in the Schools*, 6, 24-8.
Newport, E.L. (1982), 'Task Specificity in Language Learning? Evidence from Speech Perception and American Sign Language', in E. Wanner and L.R. Gleitman (eds), *Language Acquisition: The State of the Art* (CUP, London).

Nickerson, R. (1975), 'Characteristics of the Speech of Deaf Persons', *Volta Review*, 77, 6.

Noble, T. and Ryan, M. (1976), 'What does School mean to the Greek Immigrant Parent and his Child', *Austl. J. Educ.*, 20, 1, 38-45.

Nordin, K. (1974), 'Meningsbyggnaden hos Attondeklassister i Overtornea', in B. Loman (ed.).

Nowotny, M. (1976), 'Some Aspects of Community Child Health in an Inner Urban Area', *Child: Care, Health and Development*, 2, 5, 283-94.

O'Connor, J. (1967), *Better English Pronunciation* (CUP, London), 2nd edn.

Oksaar, E. (1976), 'Implications of Language Contact for Bilingual Language Acquisition', in W. McCormack and S. Wurm (eds), *Language and Man* (Mouton, The Hague).

Okunade, A. (1981), 'Attitude of Yoruba of Western Nigeria to Handicap in Children', *Child: Care, Health and Development*, 7, 4, 187-94.

Olson, D.R. (1977), 'From Utterance to Text: The Bias of Language in Speech and Writing', *Harvard Educ. Rev.*, 47, 257-81.

Ortar, C. (1963), 'Is a Verbal Test Cross-cultural?', *Scripta Hierosolymitana* (Hebrew University of Jerusalem), 13, 219-35.

Oxman, W. (1975), *Comprehensive Hearing Impaired Reception Program* (New York City Board of Education, Office of Educational Evaluation, Eric Doc. ED 137 453).

Parkin, D. (1977), 'Emergent and Stabilised Multilingualism: "Polyethnic Peer Groups in Urban Kenya"', in H. Giles (ed.), *Language, Ethnicity and Intergroup Relations* (Academic Press, London), pp. 185-210.

Paulston, C.B. (1977), 'Theoretical Perspectives on Bilingual Education Programs', *Working Papers on Bilingualism*, 13, 130-77.

— (1978), 'Education in a Bilingual Setting', *Int. Rev. Educ.*, 24, 3, 309-28.

Peal, E. and Lambert, W.E. (1962), 'The Relation of Bilingualism to Intelligence', *Psychological Monographs*, 76 (27, whole no. 546).

Pearson, P.D. and Johnson, D. (1978), *Teaching Reading Comprehension* (HRW, New York).

Peck, S. (1980), 'Language Play in Child Second Language Acquisition', in D. Larsen-Freeman (ed.), *Discourse Analysis in Second Language Research* (Newbury House, Rowley, Mass.), pp. 154-64.

Pellegrini, G.B. (1960), 'Tra Lingua e Dialetto in Italia', *Studi Mediolatini e Volgari*, 8, 137-53.

Perera, K. (1981), 'Some Language Problems in School Learning', in N. Mercer (ed.), pp. 3-29.

Perfetti, C.A. and Lesgold, A.M. (1978), 'Discourse Comprehension and Sources of Individual Differences', in M.A. Just and P.A. Carpenter (eds), *Cognitive Processes in Comprehension* (Erlbaum, Hillsdale, NJ).

Peters, M. (1967), *Spelling: Caught or Taught?* (RKP, London).

— (1975), *Diagnostic and Remedial Spelling Manual* (Macmillan, London).

Pfaff, C. (1979), 'Constraints on Language Mixing: Intrasentential Code-Switching and Borrowing in Spanish/English', *Language*, 55, 291-318.

Philips, S. (1976), 'Some Sources of Cultural Variability in the Regulation of Talk', *Language in Soc.*, 5, 81-95.

Pinomaa, M. (1974), 'Finsk Interferens i Torneddalssvenskan', in B. Loman (ed.).

Poplack, S. (1982), '"Sometimes I'll start a sentence in Spanish y termino en Español": Toward a Typology of Code-switching', in J. Amastae and L. Eliás-Olivares (eds), *Spanish in the United States: Sociolinguistic Aspects* (CUP, London).

Prather, E., Hedrick, D. and Kern, C. (1975), 'Articulation Developments in Children aged Two to Four Years', *J. Speech and Hearing Disorders*, 40, 2, 179-91.

Prince, E.F. (1981), 'Toward a Taxonomy of Given-new Information', in P. Cole (ed.), *Radical Pragmatics* (Academic, New York).

Prutting, C. (1982), 'Pragmatics as Social Competence', *J. Speech and Hearing Disorders*, 47, 2, 123-34.

Pynn, M. (1980), *Issues in Bilingual/Bicultural Special Education Personnel Preparation: Workshop Report* (Association for Cross-cultural Education and Social Studies, Washington, DC, Eric Doc. ED 189-795).

Quick, C. (1976), *Learning Language Together* (Washington, DC, Eric Doc. ED 143-380).

Raban, B. (1980), *Reading Skill Acquisition: Comparative Lists of Reading, Games and Support Materials* (Centre for the Teaching of Reading, University of Reading, Reading).

Rado, M. (1974), *The Implications of Bilingualism: Bilingual Education*, Occasional paper from the Centre for the Study of Teaching (La Trobe University School of Education, Bundoora, Victoria).

Ramirez, M., Macauley, R., Gonzalez, A., Cox, B. and Perez, M. (1977), *Spanish-English Bilingual Education in the US: Current Issues,*

Resources and Research Priorities (Washington Center for Applied Linguistics, Georgetown).

Ravem, R. (1975), 'The Development of WH-questions in First and Second Language Learners', in J. Schumann and N. Stenson (eds), *New Frontiers in Second Language Learning* (Newbury House, Rowley, Mass.), pp. 153-75.

Redlinger, W. (1977), *A Language Background Questionnaire for the Bilingual Child* (Eric Doc ED 148 184).

— and Park, T. (1980), 'Language Mixing in Young Bilinguals', *J. Child Lang.*, 7, 337-52.

Reisman, K. (1974), 'Contrapuntal Conversations in an Antiguan Village', in R. Bauman *et al.*, *Explorations in the Ethnography of Speaking* (CUP, London), pp. 110-24.

Richards, J. (1971), 'A Non-contrastive Approach to Error Analysis', *English Lang. Teach.*, 25, 3.

— (1972), 'Social Factors, Interlanguage and Language Learning', *Lang. Learn.*, 22, 2.

— (1981), 'Talking Across Cultures', *The Canadian Modern Language Review*, 37, 572-82.

— and Schmidt, R. (1983), 'Conversational Analysis' in J. Richards and R. Schmidt (eds), *Language and Communication* (Longman, New York), pp. 117-55.

Richards, M. (1979), 'Sorting out What's in a Word from What's Not: Evaluating Clark's Semantic Features Acquisition Theory', *J. Exp. Child Psy.*, 27, 1-47.

Robinson, H. and Pehrsson, R. (in press), *Teaching Reading and Writing to Children with Special Language Needs* (Allyn, Bacon).

Roll-a-Story (Penguin Books, Harmondsworth) (no date).

Romaine, S. (ed.) (1982), *Sociolinguistic Variation in Speech Communities* (Arnold, London).

Rosenblum, T. and Pinker, S.A. (1983), 'Word Magic Revisited: Monolingual and Bilingual Children's Understanding of the Word-Object Relationship', *Child Development*, 53, 773-80.

Ross, T. (1980), 'Folk Healers: Alien Medicine from Asia', *Nursing Mirror*, 28 Feb, pp. 21-3.

Rowell, V. and Rack, P. (1979), 'Health Education Needs of a Minority Ethnic Group', *J. of the Institute of Health Education*, 17, 4, 3-19.

Russell, J. (1982), 'Networks and Sociolinguistic Variation in an African Urban Setting', in S. Romaine (ed.), pp. 125-40.

Ryan, E., Carranza, M. and Moffie, R. (1977), 'Reactions Toward Varying Degrees of Accentedness in the Speech of Spanish-English

Bilinguals', *Lang. Sp.*, 20, 267-73.

Ryan, J. (1972), 'IQ – The Illusion of Objectivity', in K. Richardson *et al.* (eds), *Race, Culture and Intelligence* (Penguin, Harmondsworth), pp. 36-55.

Saifullah-Khan, V. (ed.) (1979), *Minority Families in Britain, Support and Stress* (Macmillan, London).

— (1980), 'The Mother-Tongue of Linguistic Minorities in Multicultural England', *J. Multiling. Multicult. Devel.*, 1, 1, 71-88.

Saltarelli, M. and Gonzo, S. (1977), 'Migrant Languages: Linguistic Changes in Progress', in M. De Greve and E. Rossel (eds), *Problèmes Linguistiques des Enfants des Travailleurs Migrants* (AIMAV, Didier, Brussells), pp. 167-86.

— (1983), 'L'Italiano d'Emigrazione: Descrizione, Evoluzione e Acquisizione', in Ministero degli Affari Esteri (ed.), *L'Insegnamento dell' Italiano come Lingua Seconda in Italia e all 'Estero* (Roma).

Samuda, R. (1975), *Psychological Testing of American Minorities, Issues and Consequences* (Harper Row, New York).

— and Crawford, D. (1980), *Testing, Assessment, Counselling and Placement of Ethnic Minority Students, Current Methods in Ontario* (Ministry of Education, Ontario).

Santiago, I. (1980), *The Monolingual and Bilingual Teacher Verbal Interaction with Spanish Surnamed Students* (NIE xerox).

Savignon, S. (1983), *Communicative Competence: Theory and Classroom Practice* (Addison-Wesley, New York).

Saville-Troike, M. (ed.) (1977), *Linguistics and Anthropology* (Georgetown University Press).

Scollon, R. and Scollon, S.B.K. (1981), *Narrative Literacy and Face in Interethnic Communication* (Ablex, Norwood, NJ).

Scott, S. (1973), 'The Relation of Divergent Thinking to Bilingualism: Cause or Effect?', unpublished research report, McGill University.

Selinker, L. (1972), 'Interlanguage', *IRAL*, 10, 3, 219-31.

Shapiro, T., Chiarandini, I. and Fish, B. (1974), 'Thirty Severely Disturbed Children: Evaluation of their Language Development for Classification and Prognosis', *Arch. Gen. Psychiat*, 30, 819-25.

Sheridan, M. (1975), *Children's Developmental Progress: from Birth to Five years: the Stycar Sequences* (NFER, Windsor).

Silverman, R., Noa, J., Russell, R. and Molina, J. (1977), ***Oral Language Tests for Bilingual Students*** (Northwest Regional Laboratory, Portland, Oregon).

Skutnabb-Kangas, T. and Toukomaa, P. (1976), 'Teaching Migrant Children's Mother Tongue and Learning the Language of the Host

Country in the Context of the Socio-cultural Situation of the Migrant Family', Department of Sociology and Social Psychology, University of Tampere, Research Reports no. 19.

— and Toukomaa, P. (1980), 'Semilingualism and Middle-class Bias: a Reply to Cora Brent-Palmer', *Working Papers on Bilingualism*, 19, 182-97.

— (1981), 'Guest Worker or Immigrant: Different Ways of Reproducing an Under-class', *J. Multiling. Multicult. Devel.*, 2, 2, 89-115.

Slobin, D. (1970), 'Universals of Grammatical Development in Children', in G. Flores d'Arcais and W. Levelt (eds), *Advances in Psycholinguistics* (Elsevier, Amsterdam).

— and Bever, T.G. (1983), 'Children Use Canonical Sentence Schemas: A Cross-linguistic Study of Word Order and Inflections', *Cognition*, 13, 1-39.

Smith, C. and Lawley, D. (1948), *Mental Testing of Hebridean Children in Gaelic and English* (University of London Press).

Smith, D. (1977), *Racial Disadvantage in Britain: the PEP Report* (Penguin, Harmondsworth).

Smith, F. (1973), *Psycholinguistics and Reading* (HRW, New York).

Smith, N.V. (1973), *The Acquisition of Phonology: A Case Study* (CUP, London).

Sommerstein, A.H. (1977), *Modern Phonology* (Arnold, London).

Spanish Speaking Mental Health Research Center, (1978), *Consortium for Hispanic Investigation in Language Development and Socialisation* (Los Angeles), Spring, vol. 3, no. 1.

Spoerl, D.Y. (1946), 'Bilinguality and Emotional Adjustment', *J. Abnorm. Soc. Psy.*, 38, 37-57.

Spolsky, B. (1974), 'Speech Communities and Schools', *TESOL Qtly.*, 8, 17-26.

Steffensen, M.S. (1981), *Register, Cohesion and Cross-cultural Reading Comprehension*, Technical Report No. 220 (Center for the Study of Reading, University of Illinois at Urbana-Champaign).

Stenson, N. (1975), 'Induced Errors', in J. Schumann and N. Stenson, *New Frontiers in Second Language Learning* (Newbury House, Rowley, Mass.).

Stewart, W.A. (1982), 'The Linguistic Structure of Black English and Phenomenon of Pseudo-comprehension', paper presented to New York University Conference on Bilingualism and Childhood Development (June).

Stone, M. (1981), *Education of the Black Child in Britain. The Myth of Multiracial Education* (Fontana, London).

Stott, D. (no date), *Stott Programmed Reading Kit* (Holmes McDougall, Edinburgh).

Strohner, H. and Nelson, K.E. (1974), 'The Young Child's Development of Sentence Comprehension: Influence of Event Probability, Non-verbal Context, Syntactic Form and Strategies', *Child Development*, 45, 567-76.

Swain, M. (1972), 'Bilingualism as a First Language', unpublished doctoral dissertation, University of California, Irvine.

— and Wesche, M. (1975), 'Linguistic Interaction: A Case Study', *Language Sciences*, 37, 17-22.

— and Cummins, J. (1979), 'Bilingualism, Cognitive Development and Education', *Language Teaching and Linguistics: Abstracts*, 12, 1, 4-18.

Swanson, E. and De Blassie, R. (1979), 'Interpreter and Spanish Administrator Effects in the WISC Performance of Mexican-American Children', *J. School Psychol.*, 17, 3, 231-6.

Talmy, L. (1984), 'Language Typology and Syntactic Description', in T. Shopen (ed.), *Grammatical Categories and the Lexicon,* vol. III (CUP, London).

Taylor, O. (1977), 'Sociolinguistic Dimension in Standardised Testing', in M. Saville-Troike (ed.), pp. 257-66.

Teitelbaum, H. (1979), 'Unreliability of Language Background Self-ratings of Young Bilingual Children', *Child Study J.*, 9, 1, 51-9.

Tenerz, H. (1966), *Språkundervisningsproblemen i de Finsktalande Delarna av Norrbottenslän* (Lund).

Tew, B. (1979), 'The Cocktail-Party Syndrome in Children with Hydrocephalus and Spina Bifida', *Brit. J. Disord. Comm.*, 14, 2, 89-101.

Titone, R. (1977), *Teaching a Second Language in a Multilingual/Multicultural Context*, paper from a meeting of experts on language teaching in a bi- or plurilingual and multicultural environment (UNESCO, Paris).

— (1983), 'Psycholinguistic Variables of Child Bilingualism: Cognition and Personality Development', *The Canadian Mod. Lang. Rev*. 39, 171-81.

Tizard, J., Schofield, W.N. and Hewison, J. (1982), 'Collaboration between Teachers and Parents in Assisting Children's Reading', *Brit. J. Educ. Psy.*, 52, 1, 1-15.

Torrance, E.P., Gowan, J.C., Wu, J.M. and Aliotti, N.C. (1970), 'Creative Functioning of Monolingual and Bilingual Children in Singapore', *J. Educ. Psy.*, 61, 72-5.

Tosi, A. (1978), 'L'Insegnamento dell' Italiano ai Figli dei Lavoratori

Immigrati in Gran Bretagna con particolare Riferimento al Gruppo Italiano', *Rassegna Italiana di Linguistica Applicata*, 10, 177-93.

Tosi, A. (1979a), 'Bilinguismo, Transfert e Interferenze', in *Linguistica Contrastiva*, report of a conference held by Societa' di Linguistica Italiana, May (Bulzoni, Roma).

— (1979b), 'Bilinguismo e Immigrazione', *Rassegna Italiana di Linguistica Applicata*, 10, 177-93.

— (1979c), 'Mother-tongue Teaching for the Children of Migrants', *Lang. Teach. Ling. Abs.*, 12, 4, 213-31.

— (1981), 'Between the Mother's Dialect and English', in A. Davies (ed.), *Language and Learning in Home and School* (Heinemann Educational, London), pp. 44-66.

— (1982a), 'Materials for Mother-tongue Teaching in the Context of Second-language Learning', in E. Reid (ed.) (1983), *Minority Community Languages in School* (Papers prepared for the 1980-2 cycle of the Working Party on the Lang. of Minority Cultures, CILT, London).

— (1982b), 'The Development of Italian in the Italo-Australian Bilingual Child', (Report, Catholic Education Office, Victoria, Australia).

— (1982c), 'Issues in Im/migrant Bilingualism, "Semilingualism" and Education', *Association Internationale de Linguistique Appliquée, Bulletin*, 1, 31, 1-35.

— (1983a), *Immigration and Bilingual Education* (Pergamon, Oxford).

— (1983b), 'La Seconda Generazione dell'Emigrazione e i Problemi dell'Insegnamento dell'Italiano', in Ministero degli Affari Esteri (ed.), *L'Insegnamento dell'Italiano come Lingua Seconda in Italia e all'Estero* (Roma).

Tough, J. (1977), *Talking and Learning* (Ward Lock Educational, London).

Toukomaa, P. and Skutnabb-Kangas, T. (1977), 'The Intensive Teaching of the Mother-tongue to Migrant Children of Pre-school Age and Children in the Lower Level of Comprehensive School', Helsinki: *The Finnish National Commission for UNESCO* (University of Helsinki, Tampere).

Triseliotis, J. (1976), 'Immigrants of Mediterranean Origin', *Child: Care, Health and Development*, 2, 6, 365-78.

Trites, R. (1981), *Primary French Immersion: Disabilities and Prediction of Success* (Ontario Institute for the Study of Education, Toronto).

Troike, R. (1976), *Center for Applied Linguistics* (CAL), Va. (Letter/Statement).

Trudgill, P. (1974), *Sociolinguistics* (Penguin, Harmondsworth).
— (1974a), *The Social Differentiation of English in Norwich* (CUP, London).
— (1975), *Accent, Dialect and the School* (Arnold, London).
Tsushima, W.T. and Hogan, T.P. (1975), 'Verbal Ability and School Achievement of Bilingual and Monolingual Children of Different Ages', *J. Educ. Res.*, 68, 349-53.
Tucker, G.R., Lambert, W.E. and d'Anglejan, A. (1972), *Are French Immersion Programs Suitable for Working-class Children? A Pilot Investigation* (Department of Psychology, McGill University).
— , Hamayan, E. and Genesee, F. (1976), 'Affective, Cognitive and Social Factors in Second Language Acquisition', *Canadian Modern Language Review*, 23, 214-26.
Twite, S. (1981), 'Language Development In and Out of School', in N. Mercer (ed.), pp. 179-91.
Vellutino, F.R. (1980), *Dyslexia: Theory and Research* (MIT, Cambridge, Mass.).
Venezky, R.L. (1976), *Theoretical and Experimental Base for Teaching Reading* (Mouton, The Hague).
Ventriglia, L. (1982), *Conversations of Miguel and Maria* (Addison-Wesley, New York).
Verdoot, A. (1977), 'Educational Policies on Languages: the Case of the Children of Migrant Workers', in H. Giles (ed.), pp. 241-52.
Vernon, P. (1969), *Intelligence and Cultural Environment* (Methuen, London).
Vigotsky, L.S. (1962), *Thought and Language* (MIT, Cambridge, Mass.).
Vihman, M. (1982a), 'The Acquisition of Morphology by a Bilingual Child: A Whole-Word Approach', *Appld. Psycholing.*, 3, 141-60.
— (1982b), 'Formulas in First and Second Language Acquisition' in L. Obler and L. Menn (eds), *Exceptional Language and Linguistics* (Academic Press, New York), pp. 261-84.
Volterra, V. and Taeschner, T. (1978), 'Acquisition and Development of Language by Bilingual Children', *J. Child. Lang.*, 5, 311-26.
Wagner-Gough, J. (1978), 'Comparative Studies in Second Language Learning' in E. Hatch (ed.), *Second Language Acquisition* (Newbury House, Rowley, Mass.), pp. 155-71.
Walker, C. (1974), *Reading Development and Extension* (Ward Lock Educational, London).
Wardhaugh, R. (1970), 'The Contrastive Analysis Hypothesis', *TESOL Qtly.*, 4, 2, 123-30.

Weinreich, U. (1953, reissued 1963), *Languages in Contact* (Mouton, The Hague).

Wells, G. (1979), 'Variation in Child Language', in P. Fletcher *et al.* (eds), pp. 377-95.

Whitman, R. and Jackson, K. (1972), 'The Unpredictability of Contrastive Analysis', *Lang. Learn.*, 22, 1, 29-41.

Widdowson, H. (1978), *Teaching Language as Communication* (OUP, London).

Wiig, E. (1976), 'Language Disabilities of Adolescents: Implications for Diagnosis and Remediation', *Brit. J. Disord. Comm.*, April, 3-17.

Wilding, J. (1981), *Ethnic Minority Language in the Classroom. A survey of Asian parents in Leicester* (Leicester City Council, England).

Wiles, S. (1981), 'Language Issues in the Multicultural Classroom', in N. Mercer (ed.), pp. 51-76.

Williams, P. (1970), *The Swansea Test of Phonic Skills* (Blackwell, Oxford).

Wilson-Portuondo, M. (1980), 'Parent-School Communication: A Two-way Approach', in M. Pynn (ed.), pp. 48-57.

Winitz, H. (1969), *Articulatory Acquisition and Behaviour* (Appleton-Century-Crofts, New York).

Wode, H. (1981), *Learning a Second Language* (Narr, Tübingen, Germany).

Wrede, G. (1972), 'Färdigheten i Svenska hos Tva- och Enspråkiga Ungdomar i Tornedalen', *Research Report, Institutionen for Nordiska Sprak* (Lund University).

Yoshida, M. (1978), 'The Acquisition of English Vocabulary by a Japanese-Speaking Child', in E. Hatch (ed.), *Second Language Acquisition* (Newbury House, Rowley, Mass.), pp. 91-100.

INDEX

Author Index

Subject Index